# Stretching Exercises for Seniors:

Simple 10-Minute Daily Routines for Flexibility & Health Over 50 Feel Younger with Every Stretch

*By Alison Poole*

# Copyright

# Contents

# Introduction

Do you find yourself battling stiff joints, achy muscles, and limited flexibility that disrupts your daily life?

Unfortunately, as we age, our bodies inevitably undergo changes that challenge our mobility and flexibility. Many seniors experience frustration from the constant discomfort and limitations these changes bring. But what if there was a straightforward, effective method to reclaim your flexibility and alleviate pain, right in the comfort of your own home?

Now just imagine waking each morning feeling agile, pain-free, and eager to embrace the day fully. How do approach it?

Designed specifically for those over 50, book "Stretching Exercises for Seniors: Simple 10-Minute Daily Routines for Flexibility & Health Over 50 — Feel Younger with Every Stretch" offers practical solutions to enhance your quality of life through simple stretching routines. Each chapter will help you understand your body's needs, begin a safe and effective stretching routine, and maintain it for lasting benefits.

I'm Alison Poole, and I have recently begun to share my knowledge about senior health and fitness. After overcoming my back discomfort through stretching, I felt compelled to help others achieve similar improvements. Over the past year, I have researched effective methods for keeping older adults active and healthy, and I am excited to share what I have learned

***So, let's get started***

# Chapter 1: Understanding Flexibility After 50

So, what happens to our bodies as we approach 50?

Our bodies change significantly as we age, which can have an impact on our general health and mobility.

One of the most noticeable changes is a decrease in flexibility and muscle health. This decline is largely due to the natural decrease in muscle mass and the stiffening of connective tissues that occur as we grow older. Such changes can make daily activities more challenging and increase the risk of falls and injuries.

Despite these hurdles, being flexible beyond 50 is critical to improve your quality of life. Stretching exercises can improve your range of motion, relieve pain and stiffness, and enhance blood flow throughout your body. Furthermore, remaining flexible reduces the chance of injury and allows your body to cope better with physical stress. Seniors who integrate regular stretching into their daily routines frequently report improved posture, decreased back discomfort, and a higher sense of well-being. As a cat lover, I think of it as the elegance and agility our feline companions maintain when stretching—something we can strive for as well!

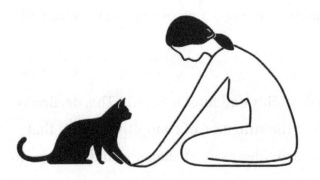

You can maintain active and fulfilling lives by understanding how aging impacts flexibility and taking the necessary steps to preserve it. Stretching is not only essential for maintaining physical health but also crucial for living a vibrant, active life well into old age. Just like a cat, whose flexibility doesn't diminish with age due to regular stretching, you too can enjoy the benefits of a supple and resilient body by incorporating regular stretching into your routine.

*But need to be care...*

To avoid injuries, it's important to follow specific suggestions and approach stretching with caution.

## Chapter 2: Preparing for Stretching

In light of my own experience with senior health and fitness, here are some practical recommendations for stretching that I've found very effective:

- **Gentle Warm-Up:** Begin with mild activities to warm up your muscles. This might be as basic as walking in place or performing arm swings. To prepare your muscles and joints, begin stretching gradually.
- **Mindful Breathing**: During your warm-up and stretching, concentrate on deep, controlled breathing. This calms the body, boosts blood flow, and spiritually prepares you for motion.

I would recommend the simple 2-minute mindful breathing method that you may use to calm or center yourself. This technique is especially useful before or after your stretching regimen to improve focus and relaxation.

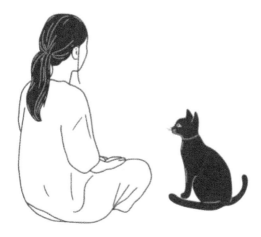

*So, 2-Minute Mindful Breathing Exercise:*

- **Find a Comfortable Position:**

Sit in a comfortable chair or on the floor. Keep your back straight but not rigid. Allow your hands to rest naturally on your knees or in your lap.

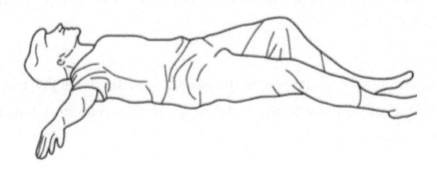

- **Close Your Eyes:**

Gently close your eyes. This helps minimize distractions and allows you to focus more on your breathing.

- **Take a Deep Breath In:**

Inhale slowly through your nose, allowing your chest and lower belly to rise as you fill your lungs. Try to do this over a count of six seconds.

- **Hold Your Breath:**

Hold your breath for a count of two.

- **Exhale Slowly:**

Exhale slowly through your mouth for about six seconds. Consciously focus on releasing tension and emptying your lungs completely.

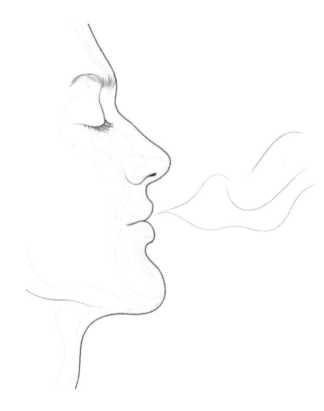

- **Pause and Repeat:**

After exhaling, take a two-second delay before inhaling. Continue this pattern for two minutes.

- **Observe and Return:**

After completing the exercise, slowly return your attention on the room. Observe how your body feels. Take note of any emotions of peacefulness or relaxation. When you are ready, softly open your eyes.

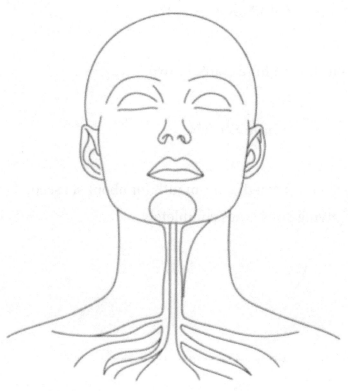

Pause and Repeat of exeercissse for for breathing

- **Customize Your Space**:

I'd like to share some simple tips that would improve your everyday routine exercises. It elevates stretching from a chore to a pleasurable part of your day:

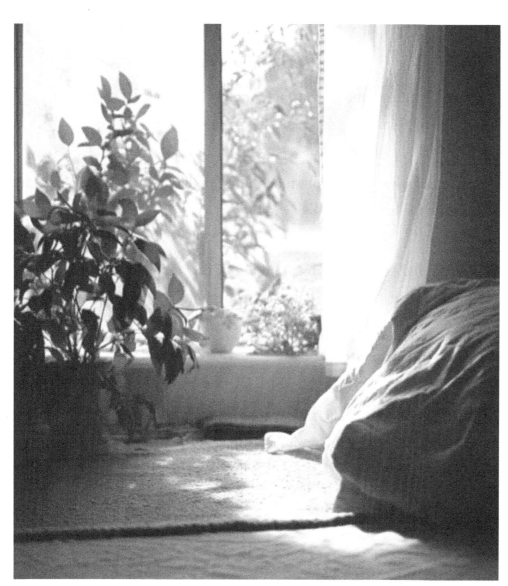

✓ **Select the Ideal Location:**

✓ **Privacy:** Choose a quiet spot where interruptions are minimal. This could be a corner in your bedroom, a specific room, or a section of your living room.

✓ **View:** If possible, set up near a window that offers a calming view of nature, such as your garden or a peaceful street.

✓ **Ample Room (space):** Ensure you have enough space to stretch freely without constraints. An area of at least 4x6 feet is ideal, allowing for unrestricted movement.

✓ **Clutter-Free:** Keep the area clear of any potential hazards such as wires or small furniture that might impede movement or cause injuries.

✓ **Surface:** A non-slip yoga mat or a stable rug is crucial for safety and comfort, providing the necessary cushioning and preventing slips during stretching.

✓ **Add Personal Touches:**

- **Decoration:** Incorporate elements that personalize the space, such as soothing artwork, vibrant indoor plants, or soft, calming colors.

- **Music:** Set up a small speaker or your smartphone to play relaxing music or nature sounds that enhance the ambiance.

- **Lighting:** If natural light isn't available, make sure the area is well-lit with soft, warm artificial light to create a welcoming environment.

✓ **Organize Essential Equipment:**

Keep stretching aids like straps, blocks, or towels neatly organized and within easy reach. A tastefully chosen shelf or storage bin can keep the area tidy and functional.

**You need to have:**

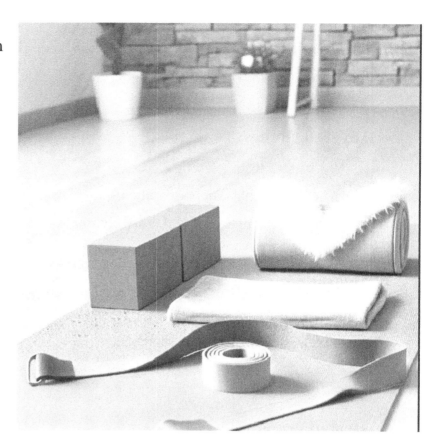

- ✓ **Yoga Blocks**: The foam blocks used for support during various poses.
- ✓ **Yoga Mat**: A mat providing a non-slip surface for exercises.
- ✓ **Yoga Strap**: A strap useful for deepening stretches and improving flexibility.
- ✓ **Towel**: A towel, which can be used to wipe sweat or as a prop for certain exercises.

**Maintain Comfort and Safety via temperature management:**

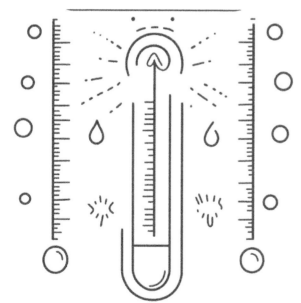

- ✓ **Temperature Control:**

Aim for a temperature range of 68-72°F (20-22°C). This range guarantees that the atmosphere is warm enough to keep muscles from stiffening but not too hot to induce pain or excessive perspiration.

- • **Adjustable thermostat:**

If feasible, choose a location with an adjustable thermostat so that you can easily manage the temperature.

- **Ventilation**

Ensure enough ventilation. A modest breeze can assist keep the space pleasant without being overly drafty.

- **Layered clothes:**

Encourage wearing layers that can be readily removed or added based on how warm or chilly you feel throughout the stretching exercise. Lightweight and breathable textiles are perfect.

✓ **Hydration**:

Keep water available. Staying hydrated helps to regulate body temperature and prevent overheating.

✓ **Heated Props**:

Consider using mildly warmed yoga blocks or towels, particularly in the winter months. Make sure they are suitably warm, not hot.

By following these ***temperature management suggestions,*** you may provide a safe and pleasant stretching environment for elders, promoting increased flexibility and general well-being.

- *Although you may already be familiar with these suggestions, allow me to reiterate them......*
  - **Regular Practice**:

Consistency is more advantageous than intensity. Rather of completing lengthier exercises on occasion, attempt to stretch every day. This habit helps to maintain and eventually enhance your flexibility.

  - **Adjustments and Modifications**:

Customize stretches based on your skills, especially if you have physical limitations. Stretches may be performed more properly and securely using supports like straps or blocks.

  - **Responsive Adjustments**:

Pay attention to how your body feels both during and after stretching. If something feels odd, don't hesitate to change your strategy. Remember, stretching should never be painful.

By incorporating these strategies into your daily routine, you may enhance your flexibility, reduce pain, and improve your overall health as you age.

# Chapter 3: Should You talk to Your doctor?

*Sure!*

It is especially important to discuss your exercise regimens with your doctor if you have had joint r
eplacements or other surgeries, or if you have pre-
existing medical conditions like osteoporosis, diabetes, high blood pressure, or heart disease.
Your physician can assist in creating an exercise regimen that minimizes risks and enhances benefi
ts.

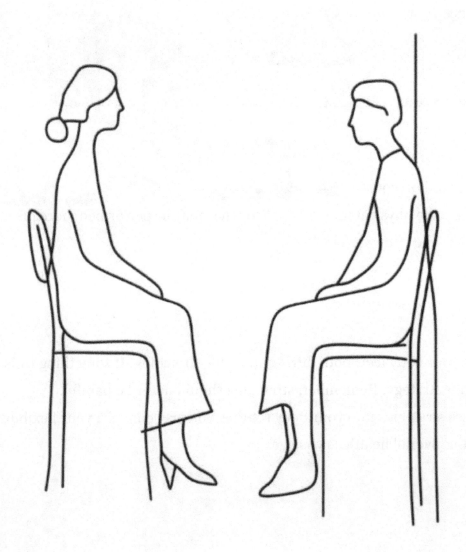

# Chapter 4: Daily Stretching Routines

This chapter covers regular stretching techniques for maintaining flexibility and reducing muscular stiffness.

## Section 4.1: Neck and Shoulders

- *Neck Tilt*

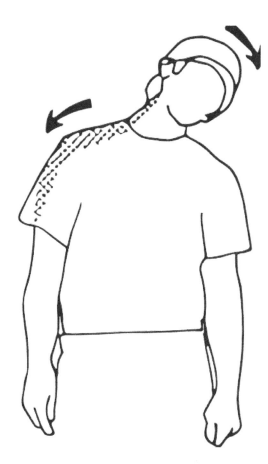

Sit or stand with a straight spine.

Tilt your head to your right shoulder, attempting to contact it with your ear.

Keep your left shoulder low and relax.

Hold this position for 20-30 seconds before gently returning to the middle and repeating on the left side.

*Benefit:* This stretch helps relieve tension in the neck muscles and improves flexibility.

- ***Head Turns***

Head turns help improve the flexibility and mobility of the neck muscles and relieve tension in the neck and shoulders. This exercise is especially beneficial for those who spend long hours sitting or using electronic devices.

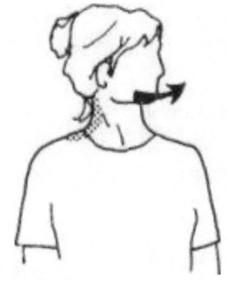

Sit or stand in a comfortable, upright position with your back straight and shoulders relaxed.

Keep your head aligned with your spine, looking straight ahead.

Slowly turn your head to the left, aiming to align your chin with your left shoulder.

Keep your shoulders steady and relaxed, allowing only your head to move.

Once you've reached the maximum comfortable stretch, hold the position for 5–10 seconds.

Feel the stretch along the right side of your neck.

Inhale deeply as you turn your head, and exhale as you hold the position.

Perform 5–10 repetitions on each side, moving slowly and deliberately.

***Benefit:*** This exercise is an excellent way to keep your neck flexible and relieve tension.

- **_Shoulder Rolls_**

Stand or sit with your back straight.

Lift your shoulders slowly up towards your ears, then roll them back and down.

Repeat this circular motion 10 times, then reverse the direction for another 10 repetitions.

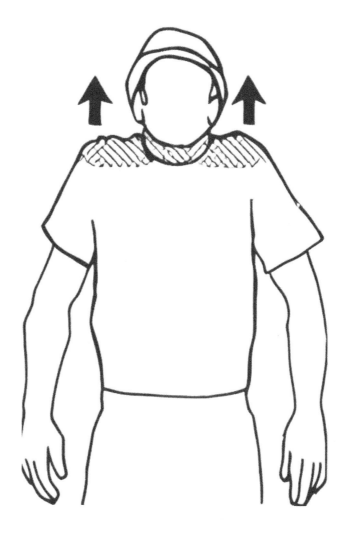

**_Benefit:_** Shoulder rolls help reduce stiffness and improve range of motion in the shoulders and upper back.

- ***Outer Arms, Shoulders, and Chest Stretch***

Extend your arms over your head, palms together, as indicated in the figure.

While inhaling, extend your arms upward and slightly backwards.

Hold the stretch for 5–8 seconds without holding your breath.

***Note:*** While performing the exercises, breathe deeply and relax your lower jaw.

.

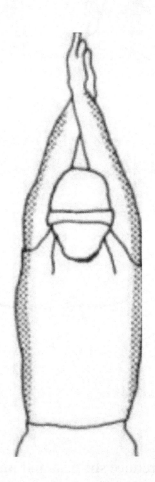

***Benefit:*** This exercise relieves tension in the muscles of the outer arms, shoulders, and chest.

- ***Arms Extend***

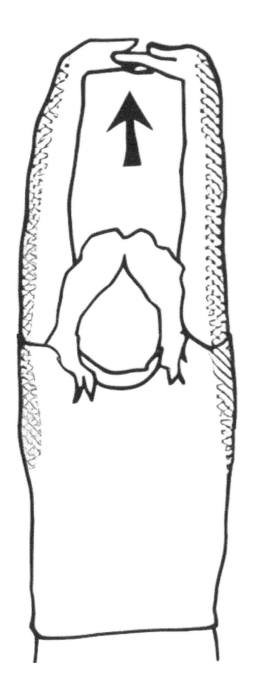

Interlock your fingers over your head, turn your palms forward,

and extend your arms up and slightly back.

Feel a stretch in your hands, shoulders, and shoulder girdle.

Hold this position for 15 seconds, then release.

Repeat 10 times.

***Benefit:*** This stretch strengthens the muscles between your shoulder and arms. It helps perfectly relaxes the shoulders.

- ***Towel Stretch Exercise for Shoulders and Upper Back***

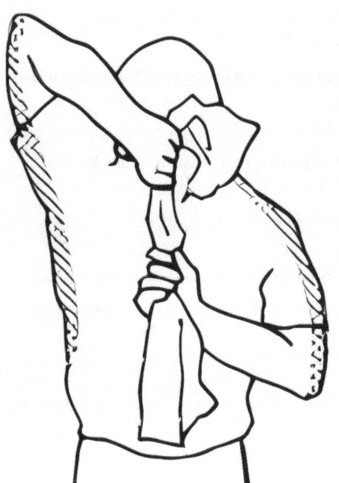

Hold a towel behind your back with one hand.

Grab the towel from underneath with the other hand.

Gradually raise your grasp on the towel and bring the arm behind your head downward.

Feel the stretch in your left shoulder and triceps.

Maintain this stretch for 10–15 seconds, breathing deeply and feeling the stretch along your left side.

Perform 2-3 repetitions on each side.

***Benefit:*** This exercise reduces tension and increases flexibility. Additionally, it helps to relieve fatigue.

- *Lateral Neck Tilt*

Gently tilt your head towards your left shoulder, bringing your left ear closer to your shoulder.

Simultaneously, take your left hand and reach behind your back to grab your right wrist or forearm.

Gently pull your right arm downwards and towards the left, enhancing the stretch along the right side of your neck.

Hold this mild stretch for 10 to 15 seconds.

Perform 2-3 repetitions on each side

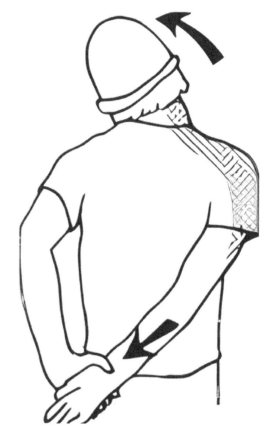

**Benefit:** Lateral Neck Tilt can help stretch the neck.

# Section 4.2: Facial Exercises

Here are some basic facial exercises that can help improve skin tone, reduce wrinkles, and enhance blood circulation, promoting a healthy facial complexion.

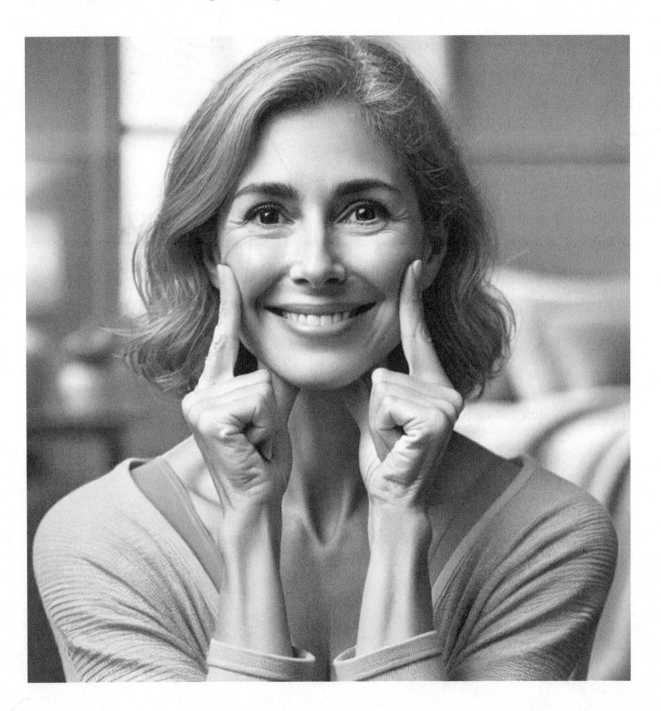

- ***Cheek Lifter Exercise***

Smile as wide as you can, then firmly purse your lips.

Place your fingers on your cheeks, applying light resistance.

Try to smile against the resistance of your fingers.

Hold for a few seconds, then relax.

Repetitions: 10-15 times.

- ***Forehead Tightener***

Place your palms on your forehead with your fingers facing towards your eyebrows.

Raise your eyebrows upward while pressing down with your palms to create resistance.

Hold for a few seconds.

Repetitions: 10 times.

- ***Eye Squeeze***

Close your eyes and gently place your fingers on your eyelids.

Slowly make circular motions with your fingertips, careful not to press too hard on your eyeballs.

This exercise helps relieve tension around the eyes.

Repetitions: 10 circles in each direction.

- ***Mouth and Lip Exercise***

Suck your lips inward as if trying to touch your nose with your lips.

Then, smile widely, exposing your teeth.

This strengthens the muscles around your mouth.

Repetitions: 10-15 times.

- ***Fish Face***

Pucker your lips and suck your cheeks in to make a "fish face".Try to hold this expression for a few seconds.

Repetitions: 10 times.

- ***Mini Circles Under the Brow***

Mini circles under the brows are a gentle facial exercise aimed at reducing tension and improving circulation around the eyes and forehead.

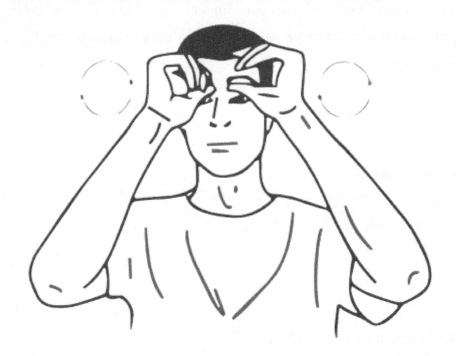

Sit or stand comfortably in a relaxed posture. Make sure your face and hands are clean to avoid transferring oils or dirt to the sensitive skin around your eyes.

Place your index fingers just under your eyebrows, starting near the inner corners of your eyes.

Apply light pressure and start making small, gentle circular motions with your fingers. Move slowly outwards towards the temples.

Once you reach the area near your temples, pause for a second, then gently reverse the direction of your circles, moving back towards the inner corners of your eyes.

Perform this motion for about 30 seconds to 1 minute.
You can do this exercise 1-2 times a day, especially if you feel tension in your brow area or after long periods of screen time.

**Benefits:** This exercise can help alleviate the build-up of tension in the forehead and brow area, which is common from stress or concentration.

*Tips for Effectiveness*
- *Gentle Pressure:* Use only light pressure to avoid pulling or dragging the skin, which is delicate and prone to wrinkling.

- *Incorporate Moisturizer:* If you do this exercise as part of your skincare routine, you can apply a small amount of eye cream or moisturizer before performing the circles to help the fingers glide smoothly and hydrate the skin.

- *Relax:* Try to keep the rest of your face relaxed while performing this exercise to maximize the benefits and avoid creating additional tension in other facial areas.

- ***Mini Circles Under the Eyes***

Performing mini circles under the eyes can help reduce puffiness, improve circulation, and relax the delicate skin in this area.

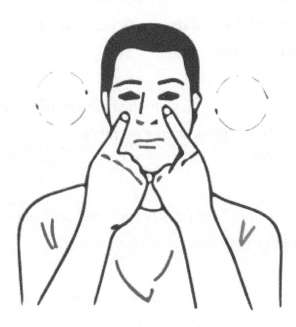

Sit or stand comfortably with a relaxed posture. Ensure your face and hands are clean to avoid introducing dirt or oil to the sensitive eye area.

Use your ring fingers for this exercise as they naturally apply gentler pressure. Place them at the inner corners of your eyes, just below the tear ducts.

Apply light pressure and begin to make small, gentle circular motions. Slowly move outward along the under-eye area toward the temples. This path follows the natural contour of the eye socket.

Once you reach the area near your temples, pause for a second, then gently reverse the direction, moving back toward the inner corners of your eyes.

Perform this motion for about 30 seconds to 1 minute. Be gentle to avoid tugging the skin, which is very delicate and prone to stretching.

This exercise can be done 1-2 times daily, especially in the morning to reduce overnight puffiness or in the evening as part of a relaxation routine.

**Benefits:** The light massage helps stimulate lymphatic drainage, which can reduce swelling and puffiness around the eyes.

*Tips for Effectiveness*

- *Gentle Pressure:* It's crucial to use only light pressure to avoid damaging the delicate skin under the eyes.

- *Use Eye Cream:* Applying a small amount of eye cream or serum before starting the massage can provide lubrication, making the massage smoother and also hydrating the skin.

- *Relax Your Face:* Ensure the rest of your facial muscles are relaxed during the exercise to maximize the benefits and prevent new fine lines from forming due to tension.

- ***Half Circles Under the Eyes***

Half circles under the eyes focus on a smaller segment of the traditional full-circle motion, targeting specific areas to reduce puffiness and increase circulation effectively.
This exercise is especially beneficial for gently stimulating the area to help drain fluid and brighten the skin.

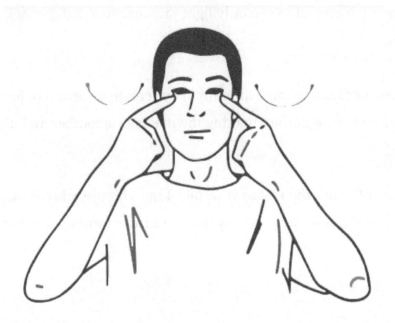

Sit or stand comfortably with your back straight and shoulders relaxed. Ensure your face and hands are clean to avoid transferring oils or irritants to the sensitive under-eye area.

Use your ring fingers for the exercise to ensure gentle pressure. Place them at the inner corners of your eyes, near the bridge of your nose.

Apply light pressure and begin to make small, gentle half-circle motions. Move outward from the inner corners to the midpoint of the under-eye area, roughly below the pupils when looking straight ahead.
Avoid stretching the skin; the motion should be more of a gentle press and slide.

Once you reach the midpoint under each eye, pause for a moment to ensure you're not dragging the skin. Then, gently lift your fingers and return to the starting position at the inner corners.

Perform this half-circle motion for about 30 seconds under each eye. The key is to keep the movements light and soothing.

You can perform this exercise 1-2 times daily, particularly in the morning to help reduce overnight fluid accumulation or in the evening as part of a calming nighttime skincare routine.

**Benefits:** The gentle pressing and motion help to stimulate lymphatic drainage, reducing puffiness and fluid buildup under the eyes.

*Tips for Effectiveness*

- *Use Eye Cream or Serum:* Before starting the massage, apply a small amount of eye cream or serum to provide slip, so you don't pull on the skin. This also adds the benefit of treating the skin with active ingredients.

- *Be Consistent:* Regular performance of this exercise can yield better results in terms of reducing puffiness and improving the appearance of the under-eye area.

- *Stay Gentle:* The skin under the eyes is very delicate, so it's crucial to perform the exercise gently to avoid any potential damage or irritation.

- *Half Circles Under the Brow*

Performing half circles under the brow is an excellent facial exercise for relieving tension in the forehead, enhancing blood circulation, and potentially easing fine lines in this expressive area.

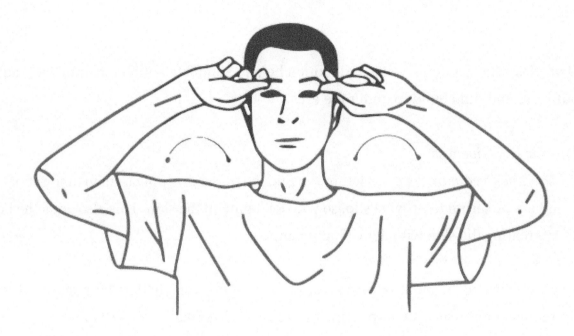

Sit or stand comfortably in a relaxed posture. Ensure your face is clean to avoid transferring oils or dirt to the sensitive skin around your eyes.

Use your index or middle fingers for this exercise. Place them just under your eyebrows, starting at the inner corners near the bridge of your nose.

Apply gentle pressure and begin making small, gentle half-circle motions outward towards the temples. This should be a smooth, gliding motion following the natural arch of your eyebrows.

Once you reach the ends of your eyebrows near the temples, pause for a moment. Then gently lift your fingers and return them to the starting position at the inner corners of your brows.

Perform this half-circle motion for about 30 seconds to 1 minute. The movement should be soothing and done without stretching or pulling the skin.

You can perform this exercise 1-2 times daily, particularly in the morning to help awaken the face and reduce any puffiness, or in the evening as part of a relaxing bedtime routine.

**Benefits:** This exercise helps relieve built-up tension in the forehead area, which can contribute to headaches and fatigue.

*Tips for Effectiveness*

- *Use a Moisturizer or Serum:* Applying a light eye cream or facial serum before starting can provide lubrication to help your fingers glide smoothly and also nourish the skin.

- *Consistent Pressure:* Maintain a consistent, gentle pressure to avoid bruising or irritating the skin. Avoid aggressive rubbing or pulling.

- *Relax Your Facial Muscles:* Try to keep the rest of your facial muscles relaxed as you perform this exercise to maximize its relaxing effects and prevent the formation of new expression lines.

- ***Up and Down Rows From Eyes to Brows***

The "Up and Down Rows From Eyes to Brows" exercise is designed to enhance circulation, relieve tension, and potentially improve the elasticity of the skin around the eyes and forehead. This gentle exercise can also help in reducing the appearance of fine lines and provide a soothing effect to tired eyes.

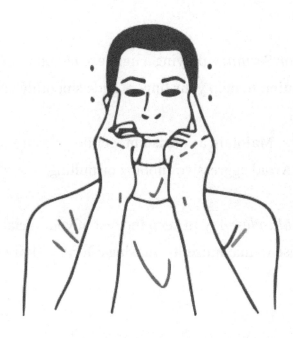

Sit comfortably with a relaxed posture. Make sure your hands are clean to prevent transferring any dirt or oils to the sensitive skin around your eyes.

Use your ring fingers for this exercise as they naturally exert gentler pressure. Place them at the inner corners of your eyes, just below the tear ducts.

Apply light pressure and gently slide your fingers up towards your eyebrows, following the natural curve of your eye sockets.

Once you reach the brows, pause briefly, then gently glide your fingers back down to the starting position at the inner corners of your eyes.

Continue this gentle sliding motion in a smooth, controlled manner. Focus on making the movement fluid and relaxing.

Perform this movement for about 1 minute. You can repeat this exercise 1-2 times daily, especially when your eyes feel fatigued or in the morning to reduce puffiness.

**Benefits:** This exercise is great for relieving strain after long periods of screen time, reading, or any other activity that tires the eyes.

*Tips for Effectiveness*

- *Be Gentle:* The skin around the eyes is particularly delicate. Ensure that your movements are gentle to avoid pulling or stretching the skin, which could lead to wrinkles.

- *Use Eye Cream:* Before starting, applying a small amount of eye cream can provide lubrication, making the exercise more effective and hydrating the skin.

- *Relax Your Eyes:* Try to keep your eyes closed and relaxed during this exercise to enhance its soothing effects.

***Benefits of Facial Exercises:***

- Improved Circulation: Enhances blood flow to the facial skin, promoting a healthy complexion.
- Muscle Toning: Strengthens facial muscles, helping to reduce the appearance of wrinkles.
- Stress Reduction: Relaxes facial muscles, which can help lower stress and tension levels in the face.

# Section 4.3: Arms and Wrists

**Stretches for Arms, Wrists, and Fingers**

- ***Wrist Rolls***

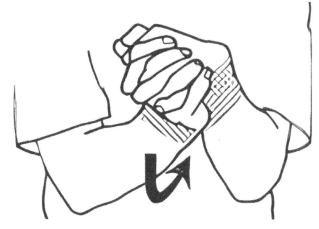

Sit or stand comfortably with your back straight.

Extend your arms in front of you at shoulder height, keeping your elbows slightly bent and wrists relaxed.

Slowly rotate your wrists in a circular motion, moving them clockwise.

Keep your fingers relaxed as you make each rotation.

Complete 10 full rotations, focusing on smooth and controlled movements.

After completing the clockwise rotations, switch direction and rotate your wrists counterclockwise.

Again, complete 10 full rotations, maintaining a steady pace and relaxed fingers.

Perform 2-3 sets of 10 rotations in each direction, taking a short break between sets if needed.

***Benefits:*** This exercise helps to increase flexibility and range of motion in the wrists.

- ***Arm Circles***

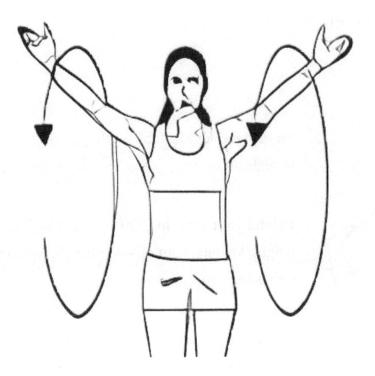

Stand with your feet shoulder-width apart and your arms extended straight out to the sides at shoulder height.

Keep your back straight and your core engaged.

Relax your shoulders and ensure your palms are facing down.

Begin by moving your arms in small, controlled circles in a clockwise direction.

Complete 10 rotations, maintaining smooth and consistent movement.

After completing the clockwise rotations, switch direction and perform 10 small circles in a counterclockwise direction.

Perform 2-3 sets of small and large circles in each direction, taking short breaks between sets if needed.

***Benefits:*** Improves Shoulder Mobility: Enhances flexibility and range of motion in the shoulder joints.

- *Finger Stretches*

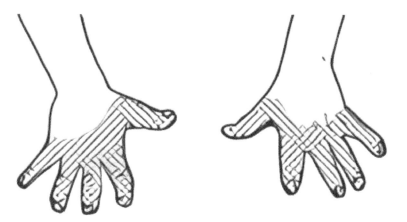

Spread your fingers as wide as possible, hold for a few seconds, and then relax. Repeat several times. Next, touch your thumb to each of your other fingertips, forming a gentle stretch.

Start with simple stretches and gradually increase the duration and intensity as flexibility improves. For example, begin by holding stretches for 3 seconds, and over time, extend this to 5-10 seconds.

**Use of Props:**

Incorporate small objects like stress balls or therapy putty. Squeezing these items can add a strength component to the dexterity exercises.

**Challenge with Coordination Exercises:**

Combine finger stretches with coordination exercises. For instance, after spreading the fingers, try tapping each finger with the thumb in a specific sequence, increasing speed as dexterity improves.

**Mindfulness and Relaxation:**

Turn the stretching session into a relaxation time by focusing on breathing and the sensations in the fingers during the stretches. This can also double as a stress-relief tool.

*Benefits:* Enhances dexterity and flexibility in the fingers.

- *Prayer Stretch*

Place your palms together in front of your chest, fingers pointing upwards. Keep your palms pressed together while lowering your hands toward your waistline until you feel a stretch in your wrists and arms.

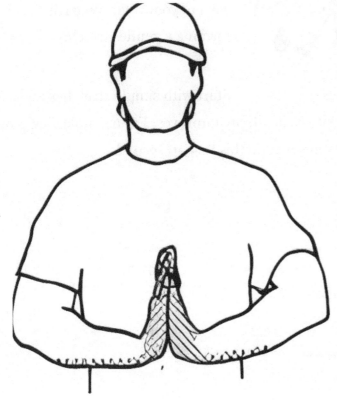

Encourage a deep, slow breathing pattern while holding the stretch. This helps increase relaxation and can deepen the stretch over time.

Start with short durations (about 5-10 seconds) and gradually increase the time as comfort allows. This helps prevent strain and builds flexibility sustainably.

Incorporating this stretch several times throughout the day, especially after long periods of wrist activity, can help maintain flexibility and prevent stiffness.

After holding the prayer position, you can add small up and down or side to side movements to further stretch the muscles and tendons around the wrists.

Pair the prayer stretch with other wrist and arm stretches to create a comprehensive stretching routine that addresses all parts of the hands, wrists, and arms.

**Benefits:** Stretches the wrists and the lower part of the forearms.

- *Elbow Bend*

Raise one arm at a shoulder height and bend the elbow so that your hand touches the opposite shoulder blade. Use your other hand to gently press the elbow and enhance the stretch. Hold for 10-15 seconds, then switch arms.

Remind individuals to breathe normally during the stretch. Holding breath can create tension in the body, which may reduce the effectiveness of the stretch.

 For those who cannot comfortably reach or touch the opposite shoulder blade, using a towel or a   strap can help. Hold the towel in the raised hand and grab it with the opposite hand to pull gently.

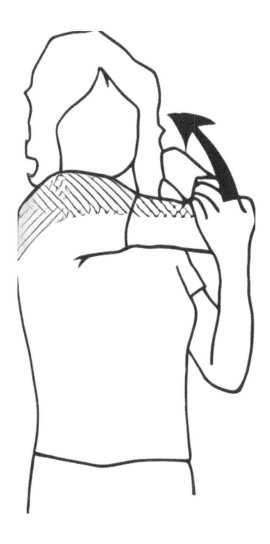

- ***Finger Rotations and Pulls***

Ensure that the rotations of each finger are done smoothly, without any jerky movements. This helps prevent potential injuries and increases the effectiveness of the exercise.

Perform this exercise regularly, such as daily or multiple times a day, to increase flexibility and reduce stiffness in the finger joints.

Keep your hands relaxed during the exercise. Avoid tensing up your hands or shoulders, as this can reduce the benefits of the stretching.

Incorporate this exercise into a broader stretching or workout routine. It can be part of a morning warm-up or an evening cooldown after a day spent at a computer.

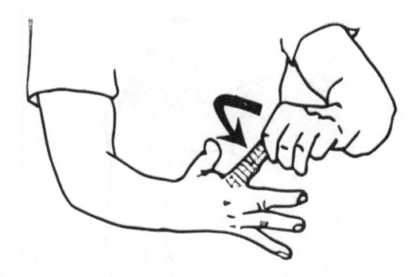

**Benefits:** It combines rotational movements to increase the mobility of each finger, followed by gentle pulls to enhance flexibility and circulation. This combination is very effective for loosening up the fingers, especially for those involved in fine motor activities.

# Section 4.4: Back and Torso

- *Torso Tilt*

The torso tilt is a gentle yet effective stretching exercise aimed at targeting the muscles along the sides of your body, particularly your obliques and intercostal muscles.

Stand with your feet shoulder-width apart for stability. Keep your knees slightly bent to reduce pressure on your lower back.

Slowly tilt your torso to one side, keeping your hand on your waist.
The opposite arm can be raised overhead to deepen the stretch along your side.

Keep your hips square and facing forward, ensuring the movement is isolated to your upper body.

Hold the position for 15-30 seconds, feeling a deep stretch along the side of your torso. Slowly bring your torso back to the upright position.

Perform the same action on the other side, holding for the same duration to maintain balance in your flexibility.

Repeat the stretch 2-3 times on each side.

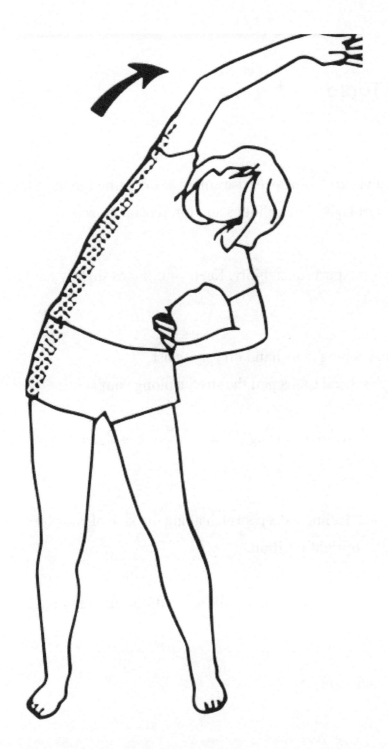

**Benefits:** Regularly performing this stretch can increase the flexibility and mobility of your spine and lateral muscles.

- ***Wall-Supported Torso Twist***

This wall-supported torso twist is an excellent exercise for anyone looking to improve their spinal flexibility and strengthen their core muscles effectively. It's simple yet beneficial and can be easily integrated into any daily stretching routine.

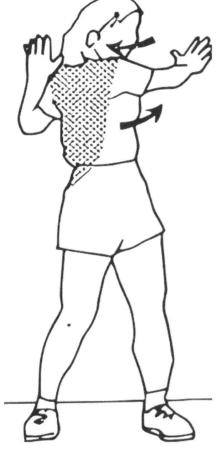

Stand about half a meter to a meter away from a wall or fence, with your back facing it.

Place your feet roughly shoulder-width apart, ensuring your toes are pointing straight ahead.

This stance will help maintain balance during the twist.

Slowly rotate your torso to one side, continuing to rotate until you can comfortably place your hands on the wall or fence at about shoulder level.

Ensure your arms are extended and your hands are flat against the surface for stability.

Once you have fully twisted and are supported by your hands, gently push against the wall to increase the stretch in your torso

Hold this position for a few seconds to deepen the stretch.

Slowly rotate your torso back to the starting position, bringing your arms back to your sides.

Make sure to keep your movements smooth and controlled to avoid any sudden jerks.

Rotate your torso in the opposite direction and repeat the process, ensuring you touch the wall or fence with your hands.

Again, hold the position for a few seconds before returning to the center.

Perform this twist several times on each side, typically 3-5 repetitions per side, depending on your comfort and flexibility levels.

*Tips for Safety and Effectiveness:*
- *Keep Knees Slightly Bent:* This helps prevent any strain on the lower back and maintains better balance throughout the twist.

- *Engage Your Core:* Activate your abdominal muscles during the twist to support your spine and enhance the effectiveness of the exercise.

**Benefits:** This exercise enhances the flexibility and mobility of the spine and torso muscles.

## *Seated Torso Tilt*

Performing a torso tilt while seated in a chair is an excellent way to stretch and strengthen the muscles along the sides of your torso, especially if you spend long periods sitting or have limited mobility.

Use a sturdy chair without arms, allowing you freedom to move your arms and torso freely. Ensure the chair is stable and won't tip during the exercise.

Sit up straight with your feet flat on the floor, hip-width apart. Keep your knees aligned with your hips and your back straight.

Extend your arms overhead, clasping your hands or keeping them parallel.

Take a deep breath, and as you exhale, gently tilt your torso to one side. Keep your hips firmly planted on the seat to isolate the stretch to your upper body.

Go as far as you can while maintaining comfort and balance. The goal is to feel a stretch along the side of your torso without straining.

Hold the tilted position for 15-30 seconds, depending on your comfort level.

Inhale and slowly bring your torso back to the center.

Perform the tilt on the other side, ensuring an even stretch on both sides of your body.

Do 2-3 repetitions on each side, or as is comfortable.

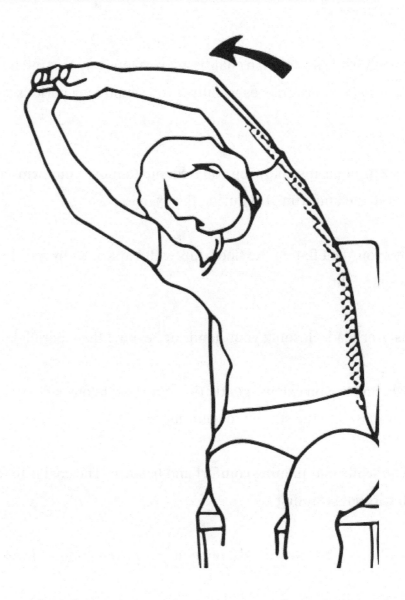

*Tips for Effectiveness*

- *Engage Your Core:* Activating your abdominal muscles during the tilt can help stabilize your spine and enhance the effectiveness of the stretch.

- *Focus on Posture:* Keep your spine long and avoid collapsing or rounding your back. This helps maximize the stretch and prevents potential discomfort.

- *Controlled Movements:* Move into and out of the stretch slowly and with control to avoid any sudden movements that could cause strain.

**Benefits:** This stretch enhances flexibility in the muscles of the torso, particularly the obliques and other lateral muscles.

- *Full-Body Stretch While Lying on Your Back*

This stretch targets the entire body, helping to lengthen muscles, improve posture, and relieve tension from head to toe. It's a great way to start or end your day, promoting

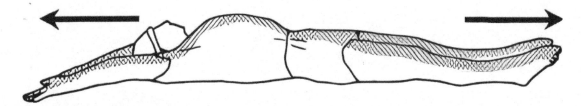

relaxation and flexibility.

Lie flat on your back on a comfortable mat or soft surface. Extend your legs straight out and your arms above your head, reaching towards the opposite wall.

Extend your arms above your head as far as possible, fingers reaching towards the wall behind you.At the same time, extend your legs straight out, toes pointing towards the wall in front of you. Feel the lengthening of your entire body from fingertips to toes.

Slightly engage your core muscles to keep your spine aligned and prevent arching of the lower back.

Press your lower back gently into the mat for support.

Maintain the stretch for 20–30 seconds, focusing on deep, slow breaths to enhance relaxation and lengthening.

Visualize your body becoming longer and more aligned with each exhale.Perform 3–5 repetitions, allowing your body to relax briefly between each stretch.

**Benefits:** This stretch is an excellent way to relieve tension, improve flexibility, and promote relaxation throughout the body.

- ***Single Knee-to-Chest Stretch***

Lie on your back on a comfortable mat or soft surface. Extend both legs straight out and keep your arms relaxed by your sides.

Gently bend one leg at the knee and slowly pull it towards your chest with both hands until you feel a light stretch. Keep the other leg extended on the ground.

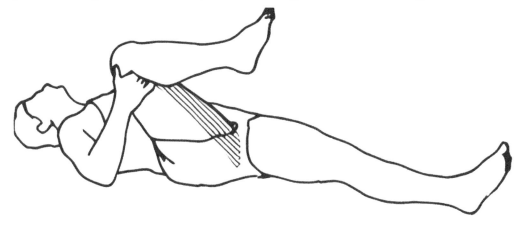

Hold this position for 30 seconds, maintaining a gentle stretch.

You may feel tension in your lower back and the back of your thigh. If you don't feel any tension, don't worry. This is a great full-body position that is very beneficial for the lower back and provides relaxation, whether you feel the tension or not.

Remember to keep breathing smoothly and naturally. Do not hold your breath during the stretch. After holding the stretch for 30 seconds, switch legs and repeat the exercise with the opposite leg.

Compare the sensations on each side and note any differences.

Perform 2-3 repetitions on each leg, taking a short break between each set.

**Benefits:** This exercise helps to relieve tension and tightness in the lower back.

- 
- ***Lying Groin Stretch***

This stretch works the groin and inner thigh muscles, improving flexibility and relieving stress. It is a moderate workout that helps to relax and extend the muscles.

Lie on your back on a comfortable mat or soft surface. Bring the soles of your feet together, allowing your knees to fall out to the sides in a butterfly position.

Allow your knees to naturally fall open to the sides, letting gravity gently stretch the groin muscles.

Relax your hips and inner thighs, aiming to feel a very light tension in the groin area. Stay in this position for 40 seconds, focusing on deep, slow breathing to enhance relaxation.

Wait until any tension completely dissipates. The sensation of the stretch should be very mild. Breathe deeply and evenly, allowing your body to relax and release tension with each exhale.

Perform 2-3 repetitions, taking a short break between each stretch to reset your position.

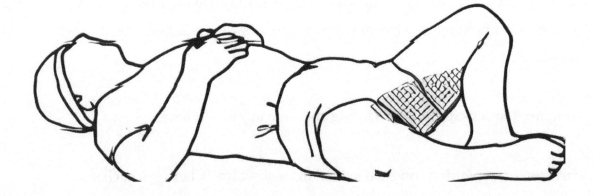

***Benefits:*** Helps to lengthen and relax the groin and inner thigh muscles.

- **_Supine Cross-Legged Spinal Twist_**

This stretch targets the outer thighs and lower back, enhancing flexibility and relieving tension. It's a gentle twist designed to promote relaxation and mobility.

Lie on your back with your knees bent and your feet relaxed, parallel to the floor.

Press your elbows into the floor and interlace your fingers behind your head (see Figure 1).

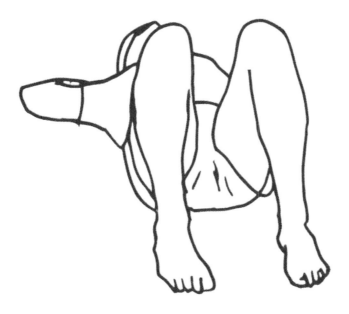

Figure 1.

Cross your left leg over your right, as shown in Figure 2.

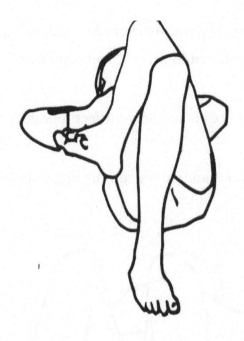

Figure 2.

Using the strength of your left leg, gently push your right leg towards the floor (see Figure 3).

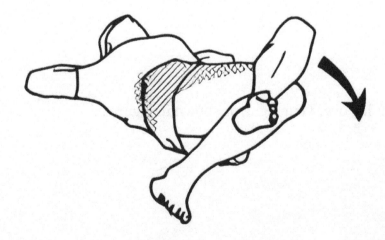

Figure 3.

Push until you feel moderate tension along the outer thigh or in the lower back.

Relax and ensure your upper back, head, shoulders, and elbows remain on the floor.

Maintain the stretch for 10–20 seconds.

Focus on stretching the muscles within your comfort range, rather than forcing your knee to the floor.

Repeat the exercise on the other side by crossing your right leg over your left and pushing it to the right.

Start the movement with an exhale and breathe rhythmically while holding the stretch.

**Benefits:** Enhances the flexibility of the outer thighs and lower back.

- ***Back Extension Stretch***

This exercise is designed to improve flexibility and relieve tension in the lower and middle back. It's particularly useful for alleviating tightness and promoting relaxation.**Instructions:**

Lie on your stomach on a comfortable mat or soft surface. Position your elbows directly under your shoulders, with your forearms resting on the floor.

Gently press your forearms into the floor, lifting your upper body slightly.

Keep your hips and thighs pressed firmly against the floor.

You should feel moderate tension in your lower and middle back.

Maintain a gentle arch in your spine and relax your shoulders away from your ears.Hold this position for 5–10 seconds, focusing on deep, even breaths to enhance relaxation.

Perform 2–3 repetitions, taking a short break between each stretch to reset your position.

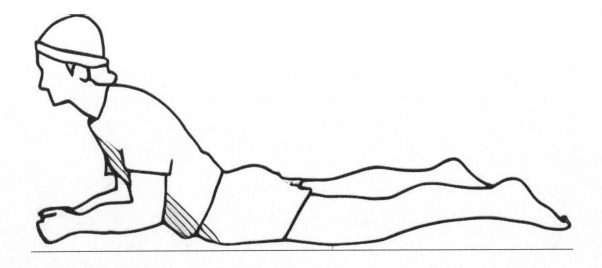

***Benefits:*** Helps alleviate tightness in the lower and middle back muscles.

- ***Cat-Cow Stretch***

The Cat Stretch is designed to improve flexibility in the spine, relieve tension in the neck and back, and promote relaxation. It's often used as a warm-up or cool-down in yoga routines.

Begin on your hands and knees in a tabletop position.

Align your wrists directly under your shoulders and your knees under your hips.

Keep your back flat and your head in a neutral position, gazing at the floor.

As you exhale, gently round your back towards the ceiling, tucking your chin toward your chest.

Engage your core muscles as you draw your belly button in.

Tuck your tailbone under, creating a gentle arch in your spine.

Focus on feeling the stretch along your spine, from your neck down to your lower back.

Relax your head and neck, letting them hang naturally.

Hold this position for a few seconds, breathing deeply and evenly.

Feel the tension release from your back and shoulders.

Inhale as you transition to the Cow Pose, arching your back downward and lifting your head and tailbone towards the ceiling.

Alternate between Cat and Cow poses for a smooth and dynamic stretch.

Perform 5–10 repetitions, moving slowly and mindfully between each position.

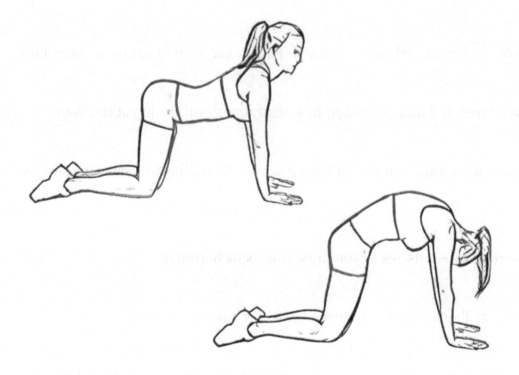

**Benefits:** Enhances the flexibility of the spine and helps prevent back pain.

# Section 4.5: Lower Body

Maintaining the flexibility and strength of the lower body is crucial for mobility, balance, and overall health, especially for seniors. This section outlines targeted stretches for the hips, legs, knees, and ankles, and provides guidance on maintaining balance and using support when necessary.

## Stretches for Hips, Legs, Knees, and Ankles

- *Ankle Circles*

*Sit or Lie Down:* Start by sitting in a comfortable position with your legs extended, or lie down on your back.

Extend One Leg: If sitting, extend one leg out. If lying down, lift one leg into the air.

*Rotate Your Ankle:* Slowly rotate your ankle in a circular motion. Make circles as wide as you can without causing discomfort.

*Direction:* Rotate the ankle clockwise for 5-10 circles, then switch and rotate counterclockwise for 5-10 circles.

*Switch Legs:* After completing the circles on one ankle, switch to the other leg and repeat the process.

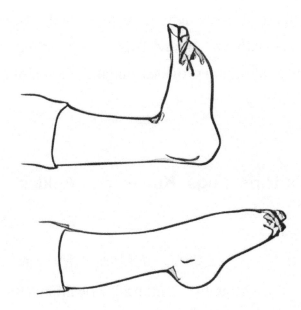

**Benefits:** Improves ankle flexibility and circulation, which can help prevent falls.

- **Walking high kicks**

It is also known as "toy soldiers," are dynamic stretching exercise that combines movement with active stretching. This exercise is great for warming up the muscles in the legs and improving flexibility, especially in the hamstrings. Here's how to perform walking high kicks properly:

Stand upright with your feet hip-width apart. Keep your arms hanging by your sides or extend them in front of you at shoulder height to help with balance.

Walk forward, and as you take a step, kick your leg straight out in front as high as comfortably possible. Try to touch your outstretched hand with your toes, but don't worry if you can't reach. Keep your back straight and avoid leaning backward.

*Alternate Legs:*

Continue walking forward, alternating legs, and kicking with each step. Maintain a steady pace and try to keep each kick smooth and controlled.

*Distance:*

Perform this exercise over a distance of about 10-20 meters, depending on available space and your comfort level.

*Tips for Enhancement:*

- *Keep Legs Straight:* Aim to keep the kicking leg as straight as possible to maximize the stretch in the hamstrings.

- *Breathe Properly:* Breathe in rhythm with your steps to maintain a good pace and ensure your muscles are well-oxygenated.

- *Warm-Up First:* Although walking high kicks are a warm-up exercise, if you're particularly stiff, doing a light jog or some basic leg stretches beforehand can help prevent injuries.

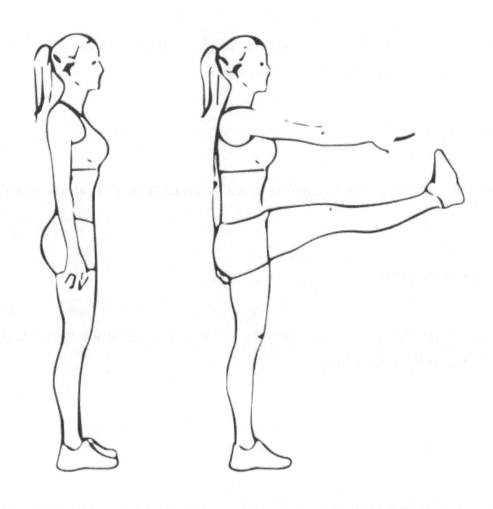

**Benefits:** Regularly performing walking high kicks can increase hamstring and lower back flexibility.

- **Hip Flexor Stretch**

The hip flexor stretch is vital for loosening tight hip flexors, which can become stiff due to prolonged sitting or intense physical activity:

Begin by stepping one foot forward into a lunge position, keeping the back leg straight and the back heel off the ground.

Slowly lower your hips towards the floor, pushing forward until you feel a stretch in the front of your hip on the back leg. Ensure your front knee does not extend past your toes to maintain proper alignment.

Place your hands on your front knee for support and maintain the stretch for 15-30 seconds, keeping your back straight and your abdominal muscles engaged.

Carefully rise back to the starting position, switch legs, and repeat the stretch on the other side.

*Tips for Enhancement:*

- *Enhance the Stretch:* For a deeper stretch, raise the arm on the side of your back leg overhead and lean slightly to the opposite side.

- *Keep Your Body Upright:* Try to keep your torso as upright as possible to avoid bending at the waist, which can reduce the effectiveness of the stretch.

- *Breathe Deeply:* Focus on deep, relaxed breathing to help relax the hip muscles and allow for a deeper stretch.

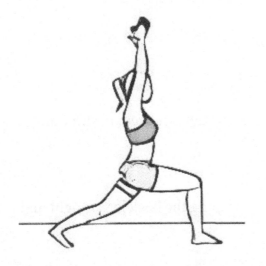

**Benefits:** Loosens tight hip flexors, which are crucial for maintaining good hip and lower back health.

- **Calf stretch**

The calf stretch is a simple and effective way to relieve tightness in the calf muscles and improve flexibility in the lower legs, which is especially important for maintaining balance and mobility as we age. Here's how to perform a basic calf stretch:

*Find a Wall:* Stand about an arm's length away from a wall.

*Position Your Feet:* Place your hands on the wall at about chest height. Step one foot back, keeping it straight, and the heel firmly planted on the ground.

*Stretch:* Bend the front knee while keeping the back leg straight and the heel on the ground. Lean into the wall until you feel a stretch in the calf of the back leg.

*Hold:* Maintain the stretch for 15-30 seconds.

*Switch Sides:* Repeat the stretch on the other leg.

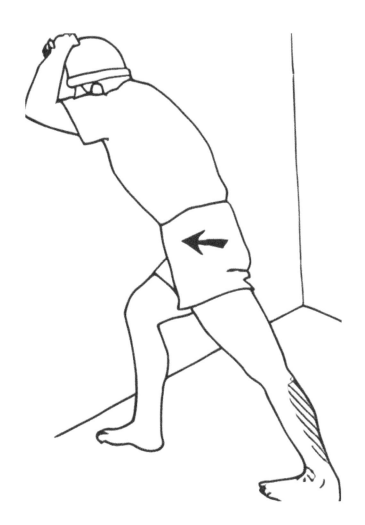

- *Knee-to-Chest Stretch*

The knee-to-chest stretch is an excellent exercise for targeting the lower back and hips, helping to alleviate tension and improve flexibility in these areas. Here's how to optimize and perform this stretch effectively:

*Start Position:* Lie on your back on a comfortable, flat surface. Bend your knees and keep your feet flat on the floor.

*Perform the Stretch:* Gently pull one knee toward your chest using both hands. Wrap your hands around your shin or behind your thigh to avoid putting pressure directly on the knee joint.

*Hold the Stretch:* Hold the position for 15-30 seconds, ensuring that your back remains flat against the floor. You should feel a comfortable stretch in your lower back and hip area.

*Switch Legs:* Slowly lower the leg back down to the starting position. Repeat the stretch with the opposite leg.

*Repeat:* Perform the stretch 2-3 times per leg for optimal benefits.

*Tips for Enhancement:*

- *Keep Your Lower Back Pressed Down:* Avoid lifting your hips off the floor as this can reduce the effectiveness of the stretch and may put strain on your back.
- *Breathe Deeply:* Focus on deep, slow breaths to help relax your muscles further and increase the stretch's effectiveness.
- *Progress to Both Legs:* Once comfortable with one leg, you can increase the stretch by pulling both knees to your chest at the same time.

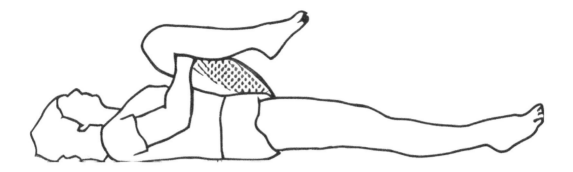

**Benefits:** Reduces Lower Back Pain.

- ***Quadriceps Stretch***

The quadriceps stretch is a key exercise for maintaining flexibility in the front of the thigh, essential for walking, running, and many other activities. Here's how to perform the quadriceps stretch properly:

*Start Position:* Stand near a wall or chair for support to maintain balance.

*Perform the Stretch:* Stand on one leg. Bend your other leg behind you and hold your ankle with the hand on the same side. If you can't reach your ankle, a towel or strap can be used to bridge the gap.

Keep your knees together and your pelvis neutral. Try to avoid letting your bent knee splay out to the side.

*Hold the Stretch:* Gently pull your heel towards your buttock until you feel a stretch in the front of your thigh. Keep your other hand on the wall or chair to maintain balance.

*Duration:* Hold the stretch for about 15-30 seconds. *Switch Legs:* Release your leg slowly and switch to the other leg to repeat the stretch.

*Tips for Enhancement:*

- To help maintain balance and control during the stretch, engage your abdominal muscles.
- Pull your heel towards your buttock until you feel a stretch, but not pain. Overstretching can lead to muscle strains.

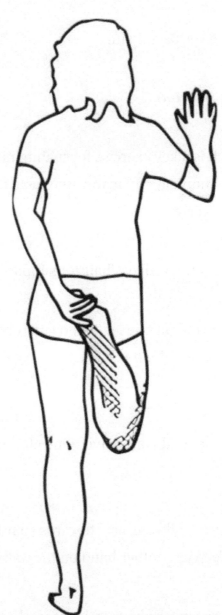

**Benefits:** Regularly performing this stretch can prevent stiffness and maintain the elasticity of the quadriceps muscles.

- ***Knee stretch***

This is indeed a beneficial exercise for enhancing leg flexibility and relieving tension.

Sit on the floor or a mat with your legs straight out in front of you. Keep your back straight.

Actively pull your toes towards yourself to feel a stretch in your calf muscles and along the back of your legs.

Maintain this position for 15 to 30 seconds, focusing on relaxing and deepening the stretch with each exhale.

To enhance the effect, you can alternatively lift and lower your toes, as well as perform circular movements with your ankles.

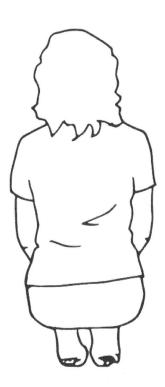

**Benefits:** Regularly performing this exercise can enhance flexibility in the feet, ankles, and knees.

The butterfly stretch is a popular and effective exercise for improving flexibility in the inner thighs, hips, and groin. It's particularly beneficial for activities that require a good range of motion in the lower body. Here's how to perform the butterfly stretch:

*Sit on the Floor:* Start by sitting with your back straight and your legs extended in front of you.

*Form the Butterfly Position:* Bend your knees and bring the soles of your feet together, pulling them towards your body as close as comfortably possible.

*Apply Gentle Pressure:* Use your elbows to gently press down on your knees towards the floor. The goal is to feel a stretch in the inner thighs; there should be no pain.

Hold this position for 15-30 seconds, focusing on relaxing and deepening the stretch with each exhale.

*Release and Repeat:* Release the stretch slowly and shake out your legs if needed. Repeat 2-3 times, gradually trying to increase the stretch each time.

*Tips for Enhancement:*

- Keep Your Back Straight: Avoid rounding your spine; keep your back straight to ensure the stretch targets your inner thighs correctly.
- Progress Gradually: Over time, try to bring your feet closer to your body and lower your knees further to the floor to deepen the stretch.
- Breathing: Use your breath to help deepen the stretch. Inhale deeply and exhale as you gently press your knees closer to the floor.

- 

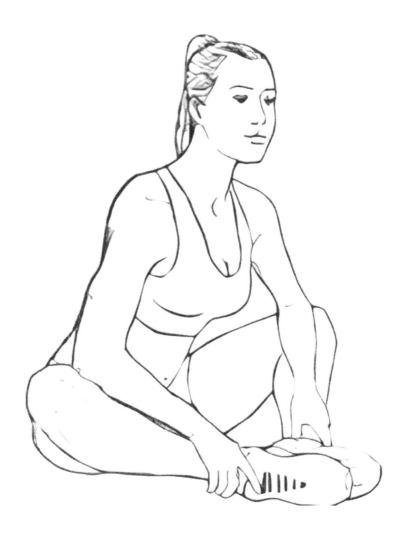

**Benefits:** Increases Flexibility: Regular practice improves flexibility in the hips and groin area, which can enhance your ability to perform movements that require wide leg stances.

- ***Wall Pushes***

Wall pushes are a simple and effective exercise that can help improve upper body strength, particularly in the chest, shoulders, and triceps. They are a great alternative to traditional push-ups for those who may need a less intense option. Here's how to perform wall pushes correctly:

Stand facing a wall, approximately an arm's length away. Place your palms flat against the wall at shoulder height and shoulder-width apart.

Lean your body towards the wall by bending your elbows until your nose almost touches the wall. Keep your feet flat on the ground and your body in a straight line from head to heels.

*Push Back:* Use your arms to push your body back to the starting position. Keep your core engaged throughout the movement to maintain a straight posture.

Repeat the movement for 10-15 repetitions or as many as you can comfortably perform. Aim for 2-3 sets.

*Tips for Enhancement:*

- *Adjust Difficulty:* You can adjust the difficulty of the exercise by changing your foot placement. The closer your feet are to the wall, the easier the push; the further away, the more challenging.

- *Keep Your Body Aligned:* Ensure that your body remains in a straight line throughout the exercise to maximize effectiveness and reduce the risk of injury.

- *Controlled Movements:* Perform the exercise with controlled movements to ensure that muscles are engaged properly and to increase the workout's effectiveness.

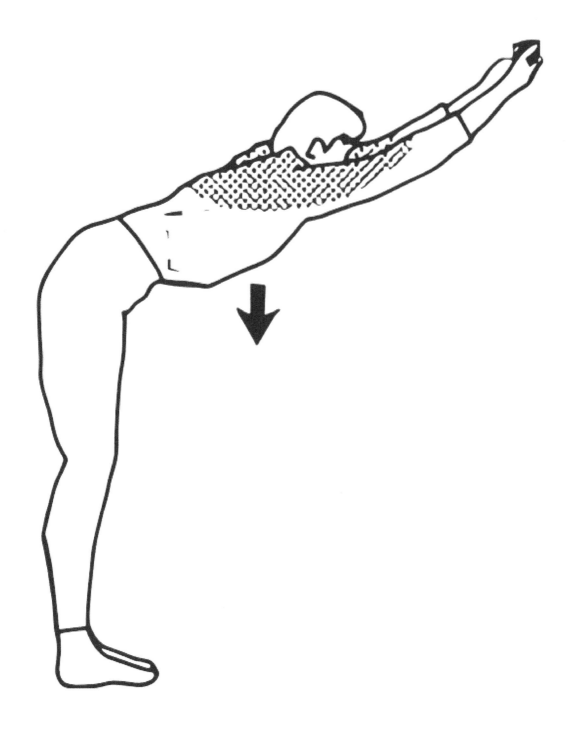

**Benefits:** Regularly performing wall pushes can strengthen the chest, shoulders, and arms.

# Chapter 5: Techniques for Improving Core Stability and Reducing Back Pain

Techniques for Improving Core Stability and Reducing Back Pain.

- ***Bird-Dog Exercise***

Start on your hands and knees. Extend one arm forward and the opposite leg back, holding the position for a few seconds.  Switch to the other arm and leg. Aim for balance and stability.

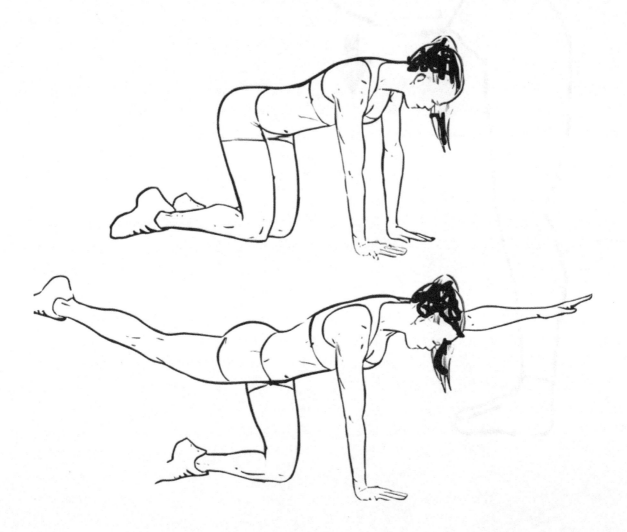

***Benefits:*** Enhances core strength and spinal alignment, crucial for reducing the risk of back injuries.

- ***Bridge Pose***

Lie on your back with knees bent and feet flat on the floor, arms by your sides.

Lift your hips towards the ceiling, pressing through your feet and engaging your core, glutes, and hamstrings.

Hold for a few seconds before slowly rolling back down.

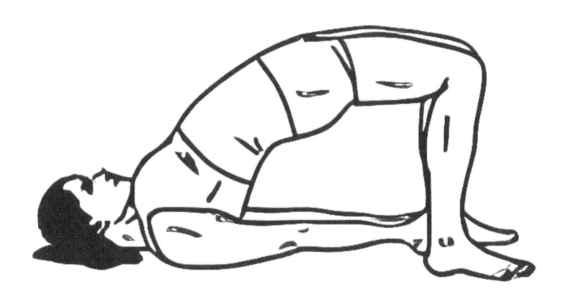

***Benefits:*** Strengthens the lower back and core, improves spinal alignment, and relieves tension in the back.

# Chapter 6: Special Focus Routines

This chapter is dedicated to special focus routines tailored to meet the needs of individuals with specific health conditions such as arthritis and osteoporosis. It also provides modifications to adjust the difficulty level of stretches to cater to varying abilities and ensure everyone can stretch safely and effectively.

**Warm-Up:**

Start with a gentle warm-up to increase blood flow to the muscles and joints, which can help reduce stiffness.

- **Marching on the Spot:** Stand or sit and march slowly, lifting your knees alternately. Do this for about 3-5 minutes.

And **Stretching Exercises...**

# Section 6.1: Arthritis-Friendly Stretches

- ***Wrist Bends***

Extend your arm in front of you with the palm facing down.

With your other hand, gently press down on the fingers to stretch the wrist.

Hold for a few seconds, then reverse the direction, pushing the fingers back towards your body.

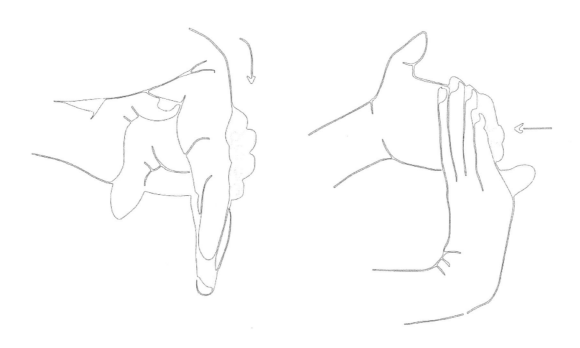

- ***Shoulder Rolls***

Stand or sit with your back straight.

Lift your shoulders slowly up towards your ears, then roll them back and down.

Repeat this circular motion 10 times, then reverse the direction for another 10 repetitions.

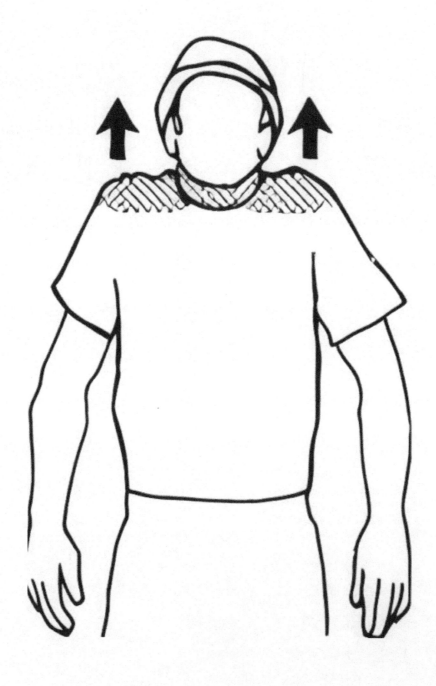

- ***Neck Stretches***

Sit or stand with a straight spine.

Tilt your head to your right shoulder, attempting to contact it with your ear.

Keep your left shoulder low and relax.

Hold this position for 20-30 seconds before gently returning to the middle and repeating on the left side.

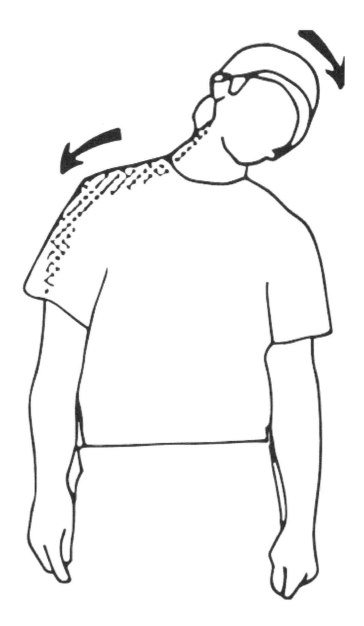

- ***Seated Leg Extensions***

Sit in a sturdy chair that allows you to keep your feet flat on the floor when seated. Ensure your back is supported by the back of the chair.

Sit upright with your feet flat on the floor, hip-width apart. Your knees should be bent at a 90-degree angle.

Slowly extend one leg in front of you until it is horizontal or as high as comfortable. Keep your foot flexed so that your toes are pointing back towards you.

Hold the extended position for a few seconds, then slowly lower your leg back to the starting position.

Perform 10-15 repetitions on one leg, then switch to the other leg. Aim for 2-3 sets on each leg.

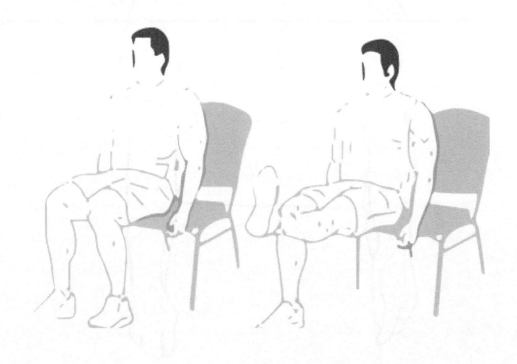

- ***Ankle Circles***

*Sit or Lie Down:* Start by sitting in a comfortable position with your legs extended, or lie down on your back.

Extend One Leg: If sitting, extend one leg out.

If lying down, lift one leg into the air.

*Rotate Your Ankle:* Slowly rotate your ankle in a circular motion.

Make circles as wide as you can without causing discomfort.

*Direction:* Rotate the ankle clockwise for 5-10 circles, then switch and rotate counterclockwise for 5-10 circles.

*Switch Legs:* After completing the circles on one ankle, switch to the other leg and repeat the process.

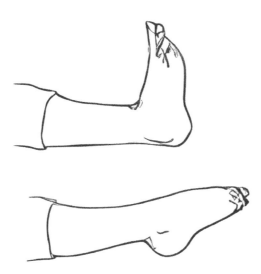

- **Hip and Knee Flexion Stretch:**

Strengthening the muscles around the hip can help support the joint and reduce the burden on it:

Lie on your back on a comfortable mat or soft surface.

Extend both legs straight out and keep your arms relaxed by your sides.

Gently bend one leg at the knee and slowly pull it towards your chest with both hands until you feel a light stretch.

Keep the other leg extended on the ground.

Hold this position for 30 seconds, maintaining a gentle stretch.

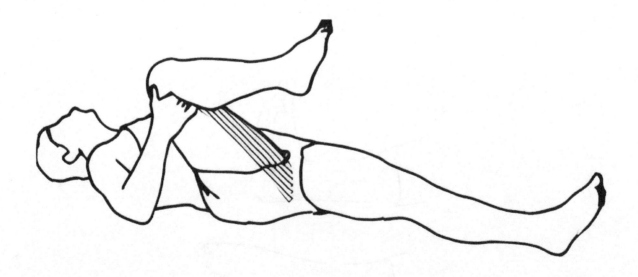

- **Seated Butterfly Stretch:**

*Sit on the Floor:* Start by sitting with your back straight and your legs extended in front of you.

*Form the Butterfly Position:* Bend your knees and bring the soles of your feet together, pulling them towards your body as close as comfortably possible.

*Apply Gentle Pressure:* Use your elbows to gently press down on your knees towards the floor. The goal is to feel a stretch in the inner thighs; there should be no pain.

Hold this position for 15-30 seconds, focusing on relaxing and deepening the stretch with each exhale.

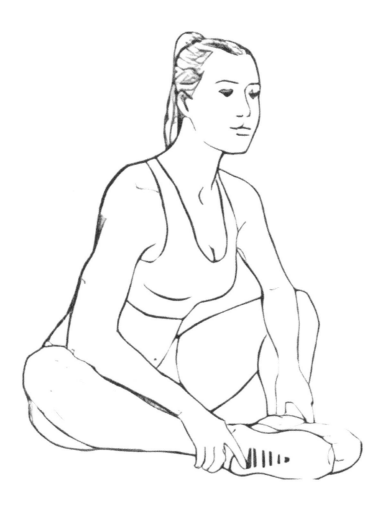

- ***Bridge Pose***

Lie on your back with knees bent and feet flat on the floor, arms by your sides.

Lift your hips towards the ceiling, pressing through your feet and engaging your core, glutes, and hamstrings.

Hold for a few seconds before slowly rolling back down.

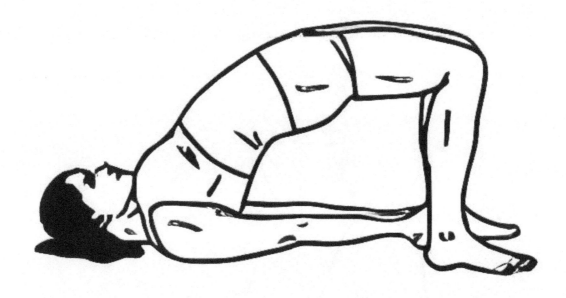

## Tips for Arthritis-Friendly Stretching:

- **Gentle Approach:** Start slowly and increase the intensity of the stretch only to the point of mild tension, not pain.

- **Consistent Routine:** Regular stretching, ideally daily, can significantly help manage arthritis symptoms.

- **Warm Up:** Use a warm towel or a heating pad on stiff joints before stretching to ease the movement.

- **Cool Down:** Finish your stretching routine with a cool down period and, if needed, apply ice to any sore joints to reduce inflammation.

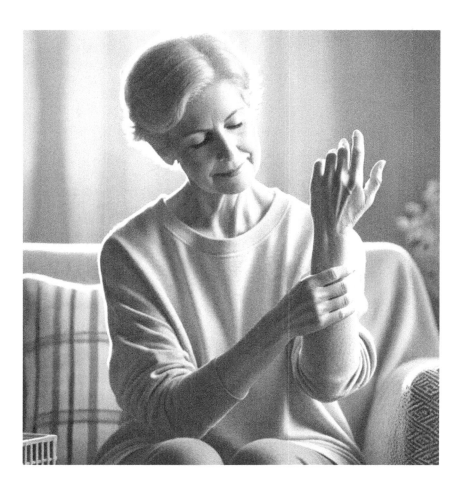

**NOTE:**

# Section 6.2: Stretches for Osteoporosis

Stretches for osteoporosis focus on maintaining bone health, improving posture, and reducing the risk of falls by enhancing balance and flexibility. Here are some safe and effective stretches that are particularly beneficial for individuals with osteoporosis:

- ***Tadasana (Mountain Pose)***

Tadasana, or Mountain Pose, is a fundamental yoga pose that serves as the foundation for many other standing poses. It's excellent for improving posture, balance, and stability. Here's how to perform Tadasana correctly, especially beneficial for individuals looking to strengthen their posture and core stability:

Stand with your feet together or hip-width apart if balancing is a concern. Distribute your weight evenly across the soles of both feet.

Firm your thigh muscles and lift your kneecaps, but avoid locking your knees. Imagine drawing energy up from the ground through the soles of your feet to the crown of your head.

Tuck your tailbone slightly under to align your pelvis neutrally. Engage your abdominal muscles slightly to support your spine.

**Relax Your Shoulders:**
Let your arms hang naturally with the palms facing towards your body or slightly forward. Roll your shoulders back and down to open your chest.

**Lengthen Your Spine:**
Inhale and gently lift the crown of your head towards the ceiling, stretching your spine upwards. Keep your chin parallel to the floor.

**Focus on Breathing:**

Breathe deeply and steadily through your nose, maintaining a smooth and even breath. Focus on maintaining a calm and grounded stance.

Stay in this position for 30 seconds to a minute. With each breath, feel your body stabilizing and grounding more deeply.

**Modifications:**

- **For Balance Issues:** If you feel unstable, stand with your feet hip-width apart or use a wall for support by lightly touching it with one hand.
- **Focus Point:** To help maintain balance, fix your gaze (Drishti) on a non-moving point in front of you.

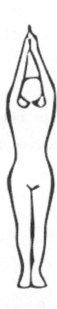

***Benefits:*** Improves posture and balance, strengthens legs, and helps realign the vertebral column.

- ***Seated Hamstring Stretch***

Sit on the edge of a sturdy chair or a bench, ensuring it won't tip over.

Extend one leg straight in front of you with the heel on the ground and toes pointed up.

The other leg should remain bent with the foot flat on the floor.

Sit up straight to maintain a good posture.

Slowly lean forward from your hips towards the extended leg.

Extend your arms towards your foot as far as comfortable, trying to keep your back straight rather than rounded.

Hold the position for 15-30 seconds once you feel a gentle stretch in the back of your thigh. You should not feel any pain. If you do, ease off a bit to a more comfortable position.

Switch Legs: Gently sit back up and switch legs, repeating the stretch on the opposite side.

Repeat: Perform this stretch 2-3 times per leg for optimal benefits.

.

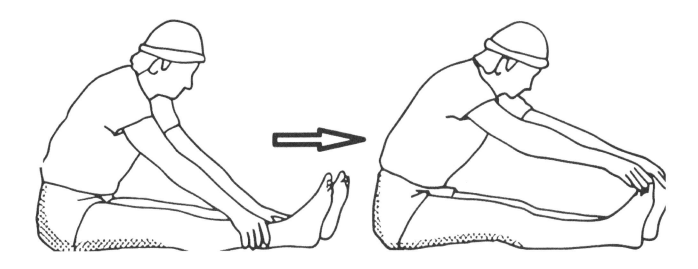

***Benefits:*** Enhances flexibility in the back and hamstrings, which can help prevent back pain and improve posture.

- ***Chest Opener***

You can perform this stretch either standing or sitting on a stable chair. Ensure your back is straight and your feet are flat on the ground.

Bring your hands behind your back and interlace your fingers. If you find it difficult to clasp your hands, you can hold a towel or a strap between your hands to bridge the gap.

Gently lift your arms away from your back, raising them as far as comfortable. You should feel a stretch in your chest and the front of your shoulders.

As you lift your arms, focus on opening your chest and drawing your shoulder blades together. Keep your neck long and your gaze forward.

Maintain this position for 15-30 seconds, breathing deeply throughout the stretch.

Slowly lower your arms and unclasp your hands, then shake out your arms and shoulders to release any tension.

**Modifications:**

- **Seated Variation:** If standing is uncomfortable, you can easily perform this stretch while seated in a chair. This can help maintain balance and reduce fatigue.

- **Using a Strap:** If clasping your hands is difficult, use a towel or yoga strap held between your hands to perform the stretch without strain.

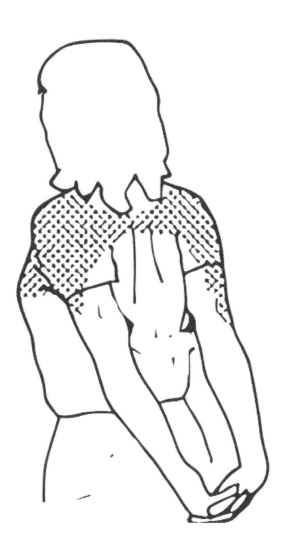

- ***Cat-Cow Stretch***

The Cat Stretch is designed to improve flexibility in the spine, relieve tension in the neck and back, and promote relaxation. It's often used as a warm-up or cool-down in yoga routines.

Begin on your hands and knees in a tabletop position.

Align your wrists directly under your shoulders and your knees under your hips.

Keep your back flat and your head in a neutral position, gazing at the floor.

As you exhale, gently round your back towards the ceiling, tucking your chin toward your chest.

Engage your core muscles as you draw your belly button in.

Tuck your tailbone under, creating a gentle arch in your spine.

Focus on feeling the stretch along your spine, from your neck down to your lower back.

Relax your head and neck, letting them hang naturally.

Hold this position for a few seconds, breathing deeply and evenly.

Feel the tension release from your back and shoulders.

Inhale as you transition to the Cow Pose, arching your back downward and lifting your head and tailbone towards the ceiling.

Alternate between Cat and Cow poses for a smooth and dynamic stretch.

Perform 5–10 repetitions, moving slowly and mindfully between each position.

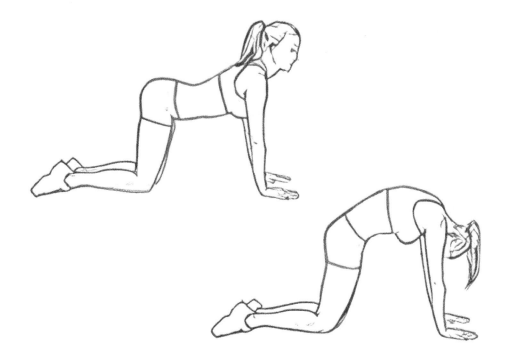

- ***Pelvic Tilts***

Lie on your back on a comfortable, flat surface, such as a yoga mat.
Bend your knees and place your feet flat on the floor, hip-width apart.
Keep your arms at your sides with palms facing down.

Tighten your abdominal muscles by pulling your belly button towards your spine. This will help flatten your lower back against the floor.

Exhale as you gently tilt your pelvis towards your face, while keeping your lower back pressed against the floor. The movement is small and controlled, and your buttocks will slightly lift off the floor.

Hold the tilt for a few seconds, then slowly return to the starting position as you inhale.
Perform 10-15 repetitions of this movement, aiming for 2-3 sets.

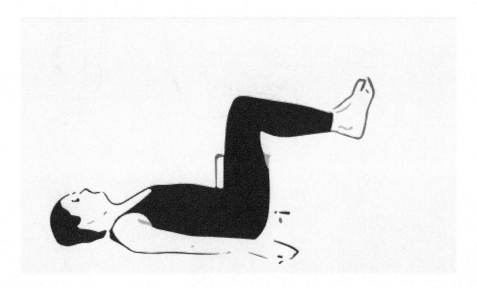

- ***Wall Angels***

Stand with your back against a wall. Your feet should be about 4-6 inches away from the wall. Keep your feet shoulder-width apart.

Press your lower back, upper back, shoulders, and head against the wall. This might feel difficult if you have tight shoulders or a stiff back.

Extend your arms out to the sides with elbows bent at a 90-degree angle, and press the backs of your hands and arms against the wall.

Slowly slide your arms up above your head, keeping your hands, arms, and shoulders in contact with the wall as much as possible. Raise your arms as high as you can without them lifting off the wall.

Slowly bring your arms back down to the starting position, maintaining contact with the wall.

Perform 10-15 repetitions, aiming for 2-3 sets.

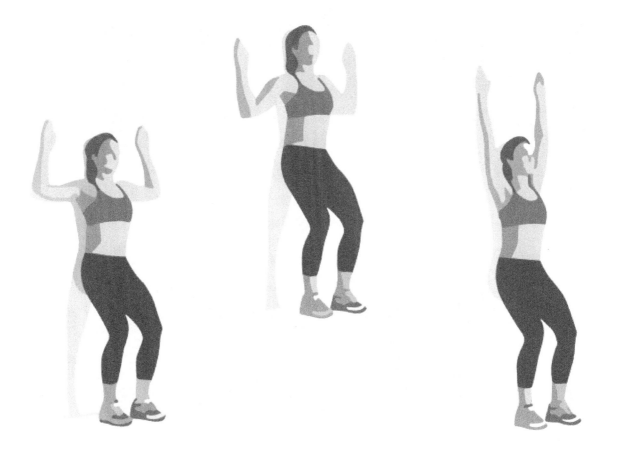

# Tips for Stretching with Osteoporosis:

- **Gentle Movements:** Avoid any high-impact or jerky movements to minimize the risk of fractures.

- **Consistency is Key:** Regular gentle stretching can help maintain bone and joint health.

- **Listen to Your Body:** Avoid positions or movements that cause pain or discomfort.

- **Safety First:** Consider using props like chairs or cushions for support during stretches to ensure safety and stability.

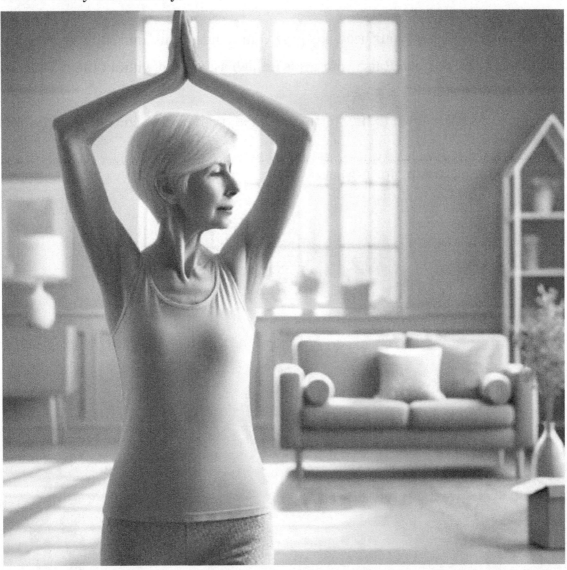

These stretches, when performed regularly, can help manage osteoporosis by maintaining flexibility, supporting posture, and enhancing overall well-being. Always consult with a healthcare provider or a physical therapist to tailor these exercises to your specific needs and ensure they are safe for you to perform.

**NOTE:**

# Modifications to Adjust Stretch Difficulty

Stretching is essential for maintaining flexibility, enhancing mobility, and reducing the risk of injury. However, not all stretches suit everyone equally. Modifying the difficulty of stretches can make them more accessible or challenging, depending on individual needs and capabilities. This chapter explores how to safely adjust the difficulty of stretches.

For those looking to advance their stretching routine, increasing the difficulty can help deepen the stretch and strengthen the muscles further.

- **Add Light Weights**

  ✓ **Explanation:** Integrating light ankle or wrist weights into your stretching routine can provide additional resistance. This resistance helps in strengthening the muscles that are being stretched, providing a dual benefit of stretching and strengthening.

  ✓ **Implementation:** Begin with light weights and gradually increase as your strength and flexibility improve. Ensure that the added weight does not compromise your form or cause discomfort.

- **Longer Hold Times**

  ✓ **Explanation:** Extending the duration of each stretch can significantly enhance its effectiveness. Holding a stretch for a longer period allows the muscles to relax more deeply, which can help in increasing flexibility.

- **Implementation:** Start by holding stretches for 20 seconds and gradually work your way up to 30-60 seconds as your endurance improves. Ensure to breathe deeply throughout the hold to support muscle relaxation.

- **Decreasing Difficulty**

Making stretches easier is crucial for beginners, those with injuries, or individuals with limited mobility, ensuring they can perform stretches safely and effectively.

- **Use Props**

  ✓ **Explanation:** Props such as yoga blocks, straps, and cushions can help modify stretches to make them more achievable and comfortable. These tools can help maintain proper alignment and prevent strain.

  ✓ **Implementation:** Use yoga blocks to support hands or sit bones, straps to extend reach, and cushions to provide padding and reduce the depth of a stretch.

- **Reduce Range of Motion**

  ✓ **Explanation:** Adjusting the range of motion in stretches to stay within a pain-free range is essential, especially for those with joint issues or significant mobility limitations.

  ✓ **Implementation:** Listen to your body and only stretch to the point of mild tension, not pain. Reducing the range of motion can help prevent overstretching and potential injuries.

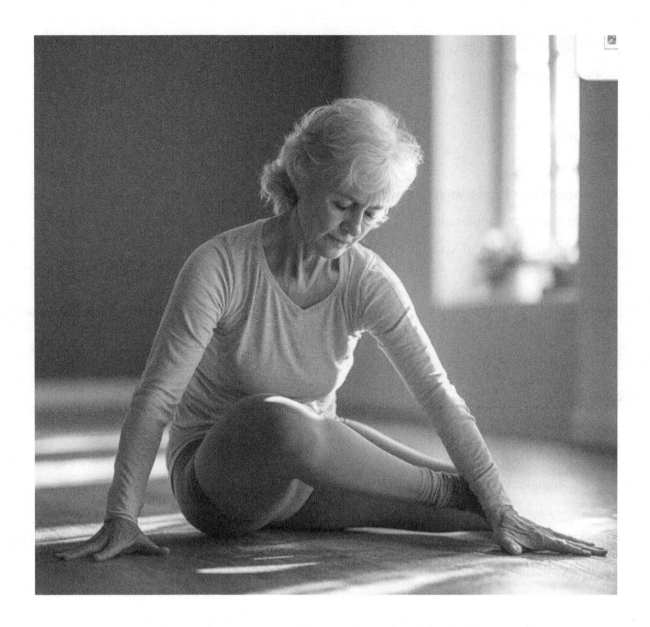

Let's delve into **how you can modify** the hamstring stretch, an essential exercise for enhancing flexibility in the thighs, crucial for overall mobility and injury prevention.

**Original Stretch:**

- **Description:** Sit on the ground with legs extended straight ahead. Lean forward from the hips and try to touch your toes while keeping your knees straight.

**Increasing Difficulty:**

- **Add Light Weights:**

    - **How to Apply:** Strap light ankle weights around both ankles before performing the stretch. This addition increases the resistance your muscles work against as you lean forward, intensifying the stretch and strengthening the hamstrings.

    - **Safety Tips:** Start with a weight that does not overly strain your muscles. Ensure you can maintain proper form throughout the stretch.

- **Longer Hold Times:**

    - **How to Apply:** Instead of holding the stretch for just a few seconds, gradually increase the duration you hold your reach towards your toes. Start with holding for 20 seconds, and over sessions, work up to 60 seconds.

    - **Benefits:** Longer holds allow the muscle fibers more time to relax and lengthen, increasing flexibility.

**Decreasing Difficulty:**

- **Use Props:**

    - **How to Apply:** If reaching for your toes is challenging, use a yoga strap. Place the strap around your feet and hold it with both hands to help you lean forward without straining.

    - **Benefits:** The strap aids in managing the depth of the stretch without needing to fully reach your toes, reducing strain.

- **Reduce Range of Motion:**

  - **How to Apply:** Instead of aiming to touch the toes, aim just to reach the shins or even the knees.

*Benefits:* This modification ensures you do not overstretch, which is crucial if you're dealing with back issues or severe hamstring tightness.

**So,**

There are safe and practical strategies to increase or decrease the difficulty of a stretch. By implementing these changes, you may tailor your stretching regimen to your fitness level, increase your flexibility, and reach your health objectives. Always emphasize safety and pay attention to your body to avoid any injuries.

# Chapter 7: Progress Tracking and Motivation

In this chapter, we'll explore how to articulate your stretching goals creatively and outline effective strategies to achieve them. Setting clear and inspiring objectives for your stretching routine can significantly enhance your motivation and the likelihood of adhering to your fitness regimen.

- **Establishing Your Goals:**

Begin by reflecting on what you hope to achieve through stretching. Whether it's enhancing overall flexibility, reducing pain, improving posture, or preparing for a specific sport, your goals should be both clear and measurable. For example, instead of a vague aim like "get more flexible," specify what you want to achieve, such as "being able to touch my toes within three months."

- **Creative Visualization of Goals:**

Once your goals are set, use creative visualization techniques to envision achieving them. Picture yourself moving effortlessly, with increased flexibility and strength. Imagine how daily activities become easier, and how your enhanced mobility contributes to a better quality of life. This mental imagery can be a powerful motivator.

Explain how maintaining a daily or weekly journal helps document stretching routines and track improvements in flexibility and wellbeing.

Maintaining a progress journal for tracking stretching routines and improvements in flexibility and overall well-being is a powerful tool, especially for individuals aged 50 and above. This method not only helps in keeping a record of your physical activity but also serves as a motivational booster by visually presenting the progress made over time. Here's a more detailed explanation of how a progress journal can be beneficial:

- **Documenting Routines**

  - ✓ **Detailed Entries:** A progress journal allows you to record each stretching session in detail, including the types of stretches performed, the duration of each session, and the intensity level. This helps in maintaining a structured approach to your fitness regimen.

  - ✓ **Routine Adjustments:** Over time, you can review your entries to identify what's working well and what might need adjustment. For instance, if certain stretches are becoming easier, you might decide to increase the intensity or duration.

- **Tracking Flexibility Improvements**

  - ✓ **Baseline Measurements:** Initially, you can record baseline flexibility measurements, such as how far you can reach in a forward bend or how comfortably you can perform a specific yoga pose.

  - ✓ **Progress Indicators:** Regular entries allow you to compare these measurements over time, clearly showing improvements. Observing tangible progress can be incredibly satisfying and encouraging.

✓

- **Monitoring Well-being**

  ✓ **Physical Changes:** In addition to flexibility, the journal can include notes on physical sensations or any discomfort experienced during or after stretching. This can help in identifying the beneficial aspects of your routine or potential areas of caution.

  ✓ **Emotional Well-being:** It's also useful to note how you feel emotionally after your stretching sessions. Many find that regular stretching can lead to improvements in mood and overall feelings of well-being.

- **Setting and Reviewing Goals**

  ✓ **Goal Setting:** Use your journal to set specific, measurable goals related to flexibility and health, such as achieving a deeper stretch or being able to perform a new yoga pose.

  ✓ **Goal Review:** Regularly review these goals to check your progress towards achieving them. This can help maintain motivation and adjust goals as needed to ensure they remain challenging yet achievable.

- **Reflective Practice**

  ✓ **Insights and Patterns:** Over time, reviewing your journal can provide insights into patterns that may emerge, such as the best time of day for your stretching or how your flexibility varies with different seasons or emotional states.

  ✓ **Motivational Tool:** Reading past entries where you overcame challenges or made significant progress can serve as a powerful motivational tool on days when you might feel less inclined to stick to your routine.

✓

- **Enhancing Accountability**

  ✓ **Commitment Tool:** Writing down your routine and goals in a journal enhances accountability. It turns intangible intentions into tangible plans, which you are more likely to follow through with.

In conclusion, a progress journal is not just a record-keeping tool—it's a companion in your journey towards better health and increased flexibility. It encourages a holistic view of fitness, blending physical metrics with emotional well-being, making it an indispensable part of maintaining an active and healthy lifestyle as you age.

## Photographic Documentation

Detail the benefits of using photos or videos to visually track postural changes and increased range of motion over time.

## Flexibility Tests

Flexibility is a crucial component of physical fitness, affecting performance in physical activities, reducing the risk of injuries, and improving overall functional capabilities.

Regularly performing flexibility tests can provide valuable data to track improvements over time, helping to adjust training programs effectively.

This article explores several common flexibility tests that can be used to quantitatively assess flexibility.

- ***Sit-and-Reach Test***

**Description:** The sit-and-reach test is the most common flexibility test, used to measure the flexibility of the lower back and hamstring muscles.

**Procedure:** Sit on the floor with your legs straight ahead and your feet flat against the base of a sit-and-reach box or a similar apparatus. Bend forward slowly and push a marker forward along the measuring line as far as possible.

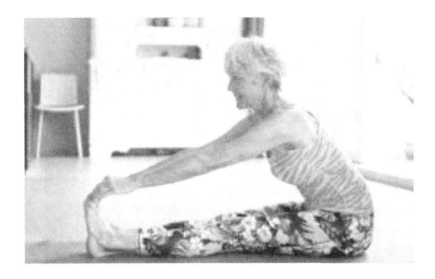

**Scoring:** The distance reached by the hands is measured, typically in centimeters. This measurement reflects the flexibility of the hamstrings and the lumbar region.

- **_Trunk Lift Test_**

**Description:** This test measures the flexibility and strength of the muscles around the trunk, particularly the lower back.

**Procedure:** Lie face down on the floor, legs straight, arms by your sides. Lift the upper body off the ground using the back muscles while keeping the legs and hips on the floor.

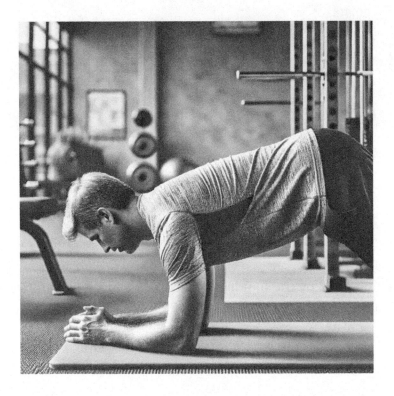

**Scoring:** The height of the shoulder blades from the ground is measured. This test is particularly useful in assessing the functional flexibility and strength of the back muscles.

- **Shoulder Flexibility Test**

  - ✓ **Description:** This test evaluates the flexibility of the shoulder joints.

  - ✓ **Procedure:** Reach one arm over the shoulder and the other arm behind the back. Attempt to touch or overlap the fingers of both hands.

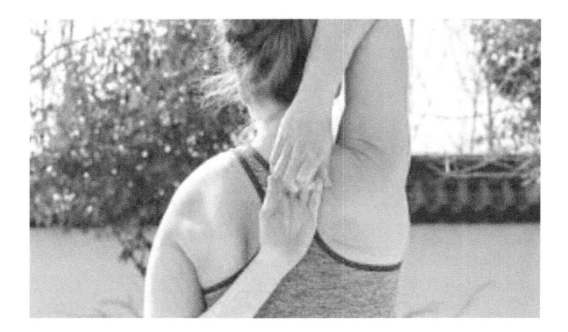

  - ✓ **Scoring:** The test is qualitative; success is determined by whether the fingers of both hands can touch or overlap. Measurements can also be taken of how close the fingers are if they do not touch.

- **Thomas Test for Hip Flexibility**

  - **Description:** The Thomas test is used to assess the flexibility of the hip flexors.

  - **Procedure:** Lie back on a table so that the lower half of your legs hangs off the edge at the knee. Bring one knee towards your chest and hold it, allowing the other leg to drop down towards the floor.

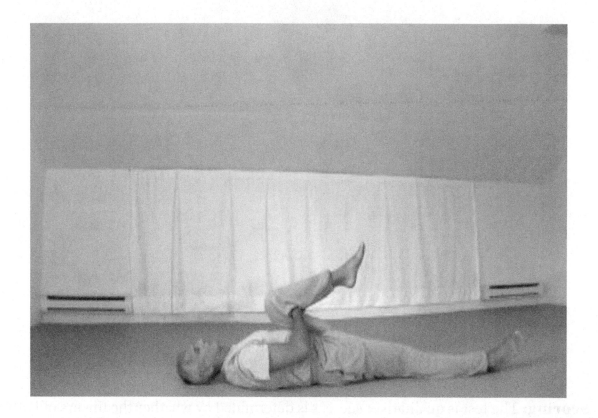

  - **Scoring:** The angle between the thigh of the extended leg and the table is measured. A smaller angle indicates tighter hip flexors.

## Apps and Wearables

The usage of fitness applications and wearable devices is a significant improvement in personal health technology. These solutions are critical for increasing user engagement and improving health outcomes because they provide precise activity monitoring, timely reminders, and smart data analysis. As technology advances, the potential for these gadgets to alter the fitness sector grows, delivering ever more tailored and accessible health management solutions for people throughout the world.

## Professional Assessments

Regular examinations by physical therapists or personal trainers are essential for anybody serious about their fitness and health routine. These specialists offer expert advice, which is critical for fine-tuning your fitness routine and ensuring that your efforts are both productive and safe. They can identify areas for development, modify training approaches, and customize programs to match individual health needs and fitness objectives. This chapter stresses the need of professional supervision in maximizing the benefits of your fitness efforts, lowering injury risks, and improving general well-being through targeted, scientifically informed tactics.

## Motivational Tips to Keep Stretching Regularly

- **Set Clear Goals**

Emphasize the importance of setting SMART goals to maintain focus and direction in flexibility improvement efforts.

- **Celebrate Small Wins**

Encourage recognition of small achievements along the way, which can boost morale and motivation.

- **Variety in Routines**

Advise on varying stretching exercises and incorporating new activities to keep the routine engaging and effective.

- **Social Support**

Suggest joining fitness classes or online communities where experiences and tips can be shared, enhancing motivation through communal support.

- **Visual Reminders**

Discuss how keeping motivational posters or inspirational quotes in the workout area can serve as constant reminders of one's goals.

- **Routine Integration**

Detail strategies for integrating stretching into daily life to make it a seamless habit rather than a burdensome task.

# Chapter 8: The Mental Benefits of Stretching

While the physical advantages of stretching are widely known, ranging from increased flexibility to a lower chance of injury, the mental health benefits are sometimes overlooked but as significant. Stretching can have a surprising influence on mental health, lowering stress and anxiety while improving mindfulness and general happiness.

- *Stress Reduction*

Stretching techniques are very beneficial at relieving tension.

Yoga, which combines stretching, deep breathing, and mindfulness exercises, has been demonstrated to reduce cortisol, the body's major stress hormone.

Stretching encourages the production of endorphins, which are the body's natural painkillers and mood lifters that reduce tension and promote relaxation.

- *Enhanced Mood*

Regular stretching can improve your mood by reducing feelings of hopelessness and anxiety.

This mood boost is not only caused by endorphin production but also by the empowered sensation of taking active actions to care for one's health. Furthermore, better physical health and body image can promote self-esteem and lead to a more optimistic attitude toward life.

- *Mindfulness and Mental Clarity*

Incorporating mindfulness into a stretching regimen can improve mental clarity by allowing the individual to concentrate on the present moment. This practice of being 'in the present' can serve as a sort of meditation, clearing the mind of clutter and reducing the racing thoughts that are common with worry and stress.

- **_Improved Concentration and Focus_**

Stretching activities are intentional, methodical, and take concentration, which can assist enhance general mental focus and attention.

Over time, this can result in improved memory retention, problem-solving abilities, and cognitive flexibility.

- **_Better Sleep_**

Stretching can also improve sleep quality, which is directly related to mental wellness. Evening stretching activities indicate to the body that it's time to unwind, relaxing the muscles and soothing the mind. This relaxation can help you fall asleep faster, sleep deeper, and wake up feeling more rested and alert.

- **_Emotional Resilience_**

Stretching regularly might help you develop emotional resilience. Individuals who commit to a daily practice establish a habit that may give a feeling of security and regularity, even in times of stress or emotional upheaval.

- **_Coping Mechanism for Mental Health_**

Stretching can be an important part of a larger mental health approach for those who are dealing with chronic stress, worry, or depression.

It gives a healthy outlet for dealing with emotional anguish, giving you a reprieve from the mental turmoil and a means to physically work with emotional suffering.

- **_Integration in Daily Life_**

Stretching should be integrated into everyday life to completely benefit from its mental health benefits. This integration does not have to be time-consuming; brief sessions can be beneficial.

- ***Tips for Incorporating Stretching***
  - **Set realistic goals**:

Start with just a few minutes a day and gradually increase the duration as your flexibility improves.

  - **Create a routine**:

Try to stretch at the same time each day to establish it as a habit.

  - **Mix it up**:

Incorporate a variety of stretching techniques to keep the routine interesting and engaging.

So,

Stretching has several mental advantages and can considerably improve one's quality of life. Stretching is an effective mental health aid because it reduces stress, improves mood, increases attention, and promotes better sleep. Stretching is expected to become a fundamental part of everyday routines as more people discover and accept its advantages, not just for physical but also for mental well-being. Stretching, whether as a stand-alone activity or as part of a larger workout routine, is a simple and accessible technique to assist both the mind and body.

# Conclusion

Maintaining flexibility and general fitness as we age is critical to ensure quality of life and independence. Stretching and other physical exercises daily are not only healthy but also necessary for those over the age of 50. The path to better health and flexibility necessitates persistence and motivation, traits that can change the aging process into a more lively and active stage of life.

Developing a regimen that incorporates regular flexibility exercises can result in considerable gain sin mobility, pain relief, and overall well-being.

The goal is to stay dedicated and make these exercises part of your everyday routine. Remember, it's never too late to begin, and the benefits of starting now will have long-term effects on your health and mobility.

Alison Poole advises all readers to embark on this journey with a positive outlook and resolve. Establish achievable goals, monitor your improvements, and take pride in all your accomplishments, even the minor ones.

Include a diverse array of exercises in your regimen and gather support from friends or community groups to keep your routine captivating and enjoyable. Let the success stories of others who have enhanced their flexibility and health motivate you to persevere.

You may enjoy your favorite hobbies and live an active life for years to come if you prioritize your health and stay motivated. So, take the first step now and continue with confidence, knowing that each stretch and effort puts you closer to becoming healthier and more flexible.
By committing to these simple exercises, you can significantly improve your quality of life, feeling younger and more energetic.

If you've found value in these routines, I would appreciate it if you consider sharing your thoughts with a review on Amazon.
Your feedback can inspire others to start their journey towards better health and vitality.

# Chapter 9: Additional Resources

## Your journal (example):

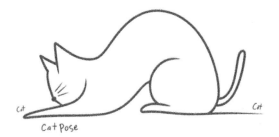

Cat Pose

*Stretching Journal Entry: _____*

*General Information:*

- *Date: _____*
- *Time of Day: Morning*
- *Duration: 10 minutes*

*Physical Conditions:*

- *Initial Body Feelings: Felt slightly stiff in the lower back and hamstrings from sitting at the desk yesterday.*

*Energy Level: Medium*

*Stretching Routine:*

- *Hamstring Stretch*

*Duration: 5 minutes (2.5 minutes each leg)*

*Technique: Seated on the floor, reached toward toes with a straight back.*

*Intensity: Moderate; used a yoga strap to aid reaching further.*

*Notes: Felt a good stretch, slight discomfort but no pain.*

- *Cat-Cow Stretch*

*Duration: 3 minutes*

*Repetitions: 10 slow rounds*

*Intensity: Light*

*Notes: Helped alleviate some stiffness in the lower back.*

- *Chest Opener*

*Duration: 2 minutes*

*Technique: Used a door frame to stretch the chest muscles.*

*Intensity: Moderate*

*Notes: Felt a relieving stretch across the chest and shoulders.*

- *Goals for Today's Session:*

*Objective: Focus on alleviating lower back stiffness and improving hamstring flexibility.*

*Achievement: Successfully used the strap for a deeper hamstring stretch and felt less stiff in the back post-session.*

- *Reflections:*

*Feelings Post-Session: More relaxed and flexible; the back feels looser.*

*Challenges: Hamstrings still feel a bit tight; need to possibly increase hold time or frequency.*

*Successes: Managed to stretch deeper than last week using the yoga strap.*

- *Adjustments for Next Session:*

*Plan: Increase hamstring stretch hold time to 3 minutes each leg.*

*Motivational Note: Great job today! Remember, progress is a slow and steady journey. Keep focusing on small improvements.*

*Visual Progress Tracking:*

*Photo Attached: None today.*

*Flexibility Measurement: Reached 2 inches closer to the toes than at the start of the month.*

# Disclaimer

The information provided in this book is for educational and informational purposes only and is not intended as a substitute for advice from your physician or other healthcare professional. You should not use the information in this book for diagnosis or treatment of any health problem or for prescription of any medication or other treatment. You should consult with a healthcare professional before starting any diet, exercise, or supplementation program, before taking any medication, or if you have or suspect you might have a health problem. The author and publisher of this book are not responsible for any adverse effects or consequences resulting from the use of any suggestions, preparations, or methods described in this book. The use of the information in this book is strictly at your own risk.

Made in United States
Orlando, FL
23 September 2024

51837460R00070